Freedom from Disease

Also by Peter Morgan Kash

Make Your Own Luck

Also by Jay Lombard, D.O.

The Brain Wellness Plan
Balance Your Brain, Balance Your Life

Freedom
from Disease

———————•———————

The Breakthrough Approach
to Preventing Cancer,
Heart Disease, Alzheimer's,
and Depression by
Controlling Insulin

———————•———————

PETER MORGAN KASH
and JAY LOMBARD, D.O.,
with TOM MONTE

ST. MARTIN'S PRESS 〽 NEW YORK

www.stmartins.com

Library of Congress Cataloging-in-Publication Data

Kash, Peter Morgan.
Freedom from disease : the breakthrough approach to preventing
cancer, heart disease, Alzheimer's, and depression by controlling insulin /
by Peter Morgan Kash and Jay Lombard with Tom Monte.
p.   cm.
ISBN-13: 978-0-312-35869-3
ISBN-10: 0-312-35869-5
1. Insulin resistance—Popular works.   2. Metabolic syndrome—
Popular works.   3. Chronic diseases—Prevention.   I. Lombard,
Jay.   II. Monte, Tom.   III. Title.
RC662.4.K373 2008
615'.365—dc22
2008010386

10 9 8 7 6 5 4 3 2

Note to Reader

———•———

This book is for informational purposes only. It is not intended to take the place of medical advice from a trained medical professional. Readers are advised to consult a physician or other qualified health professional regarding diet and exercise or before acting on any of the information in this book.

Contents

———•———

———

Contents

Acknowledgments

PETER KASH

First and foremost, I want to thank my coauthors, Dr. Jay Lombard and Tom Monte, who share my vision on helping end disease through health consciousness and science education. Thank you to Toby Monte for supplying delicious and nutritious recipes. My deepest gratitude to our agent, Jim Levine, who has been steadfast in sharing our book, and to our editor, Sheila Curry Oakes, whose perseverance brought out the best in us. Thank you to Alyse Diamond, our assistant editor, for all of her patience.

I need to thank my partners, David Tanen and Joshua Kazam, for their unrelenting support and patience in all of my endeavors. My thanks to Dr. Paul Bolno, Dr. David Lau, Ben Bernstein, Chris Wilfong, Steve Blum, Tim McInerney, Tyana Kurtz, Scott Navins, and the whole Two River team, especially Pete VanDyk. The book would not have been possible without the aid of my executive assistant, Susan Convery.

A special thanks to Dr. Mehmet Oz, for his words of vision, and his guidance and encouragement throughout the process.

The following doctors have taught me selflessness in trying to make the world a better place through their gifts in medicine and science: Bradley Artel, Todd Ashkenaz, Henry Baraket, Yoni Barnhard, Arie Belldegrun, Greg Berkowitz, Peter Blauzvern, Steven Blechman, Paul Bunn, Dan Carr, Jeffrey Dacher, T. Forcht Dagi, Peer Dar, Jim Giglio, Scott Bernstein, Mark and Francine Einstein, Israel Franco, Scott Fields, Jacob Gottlieb, David Guyer, Joshua Fogelman, Silviu Itescu, Bonnie Kazam, Ezra Kazam, Elias Kazam, Howard Kessler, Robert Klein, Barry Kraushaar, Robert Langer, Ilan Lapidot, Adel Mansour, Michael Mashaal, Fred Mermelstein, Chris Michelsen, Edmundo Muniz, Siu Ping Negrin, Binh Nguyen, Larry Norton, Ron Nutovitz, Ken Pearlman, Nanci Pittman, Mark Rachesky, Gregg Rockower, Alicia Romano, Eric Rose, Jeff Schnapper, Mark Seem, Ariel Sherbany, Gary Stein, Bart Silverman, Ellen Strahlman, Lester Wold, Curtis Wright, and William Zinn.

I also wish to thank Dr. Schnall, Dr. Goldberg, Dr. Pelcovitz, and Dr. Sokolow, for their guidance and patience.

After witnessing the strength of my mother during her bout with type II diabetes, I have yet to meet anyone with a stronger will to survive. May this book help to prevent anyone else from experiencing the pain and anguish that she endured.

Lastly, I want to thank my wife and best friend, Donna, who encourages me to reach new heights, and our four children, Jared, Colby, Shantal, and Zena, who make it all worthwhile. I hope that this book helps their generation lead healthier, happier lives.

JAY LOMBARD

First, to Peter Kash, my very close friend, whose tenacity and persistence made this book possible. To James Levine, the best agent in the business. To Tom Monte, for his incredible ability to synthesize difficult medical concepts and make them explainable. To Sheila Curry Oakes, for her phenomenal editorial guidance. To Jeff Bland, for providing the inspiration to change the medical landscape. To Mehmet Oz, for being an incredible friend, teacher, and physician. To Sridhar Chilimuri, for being one of the best role models and leaders in his guidance of the medicine department at Bronx-Lebanon Hospital. Most important, I would like to thank my beautiful wife, Rita, and my daughters, Julie and Sofia, for their love and laughter and for making it all worthwhile.

Foreword

———•———

We Stand on the Precipice

Our society's emphasis upon treating disease, as opposed to keeping people well, has just about run its course. In the relatively near future, our medical system, along with wide swaths of the American economy, will either be bankrupt or on the road to recovery. That's the crucial fork in the road that we will face in the twenty-first century. If the medical system goes bankrupt, our society will face widespread chaos. If we learn from our mistakes, we will evolve into a more sustainable, healthier culture. Individually, each of us will enjoy well-being—and all that that means—along with greater freedom from pharmaceutical drugs and avoidable medical procedures. Collectively, our society will be more creative and thus better able to direct our considerable resources toward other problems we currently face. As with every species, there are times when the conditions demand an evolutionary leap. Humanity now faces one of those times.

Essentially, our challenge is to change behaviors that have become a threat to our health and our ability to deliver medical services to all our people. The foods most of us are eating today and our lack of physical activity are poisoning our bodies and altering the way our central nervous systems function, thus causing a wide array of physical and mental disorders, as well as premature death.

As a professor and vice chair of surgery at New York-Presbyterian/Columbia University Medical Center, I see the effects of these behaviors every day in my medical practice and in the operating room. The sludge-filled coronary arteries, diseased gall bladders, fatty livers, hypertension-scarred kidneys, and cancerous tumors are just some of the consequences of our toxic lifestyle. Unbeknownst to most of us, so, too, are many of the mood and brain disorders that so many of us suffer from today.

Our health care system addresses the multiple epidemics we face by treating illness after it arises, rather than address the causes of disease at their source. Not surprisingly, medicine cannot keep pace with the rising rates of illness because we are treating people at the wrong end of the problem.

A great many of the diseases we face today arise from our inability to manage our weight, with more than two-thirds of Americans overweight, and more than a third obese. During the 1980s, little more than a third of Americans were overweight and only 15 percent were obese.

Similar disease patterns are emerging around the world. The World Health Organization has stated that more than one billion people worldwide are overweight and about 300 million are now obese. Almost unbelievably, those who are overweight now outnumber those who are undernourished (there are now about 600 million hungry people worldwide).

The problem with overweight and obesity is that they have a domino effect on our biology. We don't just get fat. Overweight changes our internal chemistry so that the basic commands that are passed between cells, and within them, are dramatically altered. Soon, this misinformation causes genes to malfunction, which in turn cause an array of illnesses, including diabetes, high blood pressure, heart disease, mood disorders, Alzheimer's disease, and many common cancers.

Obesity's partner in crime, diabetes, is now a worldwide epidemic. There are more than twenty million diabetics in the United States today. By 2025, that number will likely double. By the year 2050, the number of people worldwide with diabetes will reach 250 million unless something is done to stop this raging epidemic. As with overweight, diabetes causes the widespread breakdown of health, raising the risk of infection, gangrene, amputation, blindness, kidney disorders, and heart attack.

In the past, illnesses such as diabetes and heart disease were considered diseases of old age, but all of that is changing. Today, we are seeing an ever-increasing number of children who are overweight, diabetic, and suffering from the early stages of heart disease—all ominous signs for our future.

Needless to say, treating these illnesses costs inconceivable sums of money. Today, annual health care costs in the United States hover at about two trillion dollars, two and a half times what they were in 1990, and seven times what they were in 1980. The vast majority of this money is being spent on catastrophic care, especially the medical treatment received at the end of life. Half of the total health care bill for treating the average American over the course of his or her lifetime will be spent during that person's final eight years of life. If things continue as they are going, the emergence of the baby boomers into old age—along with the multiple epidemics they'll suffer from—will crush our health care system. Unless something is done to improve our overall health, our society may be forced to limit medical care in order to curtail costs. Eventually, many will be shut out of the health care system, leaving increasing numbers of us sick and untreated. Such a reality would have a catastrophic effect on our society.

TURNING THINGS AROUND

The question is, What can we do about it? Peter Kash, Jay Lombard, and Tom Monte have provided a penetrating analysis of what's going wrong in the human body, and what we all can do to restore our health. As their insightful book shows, overweight, diabetes, heart disease, Alzheimer's, many mood disorders, and common forms of cancer may stem from the same underlying root cause. That cause is insulin resistance.

Insulin, a hormone produced by the body that allows blood sugar to enter cells and be utilized as fuel, is a key regulator that determines health and illness for most of us today. When we eat foods that drive insulin levels up, and keep them elevated, cellular function is altered and cells behave in aberrant ways, thus forming the basis for many of the diseases we face today.

How does insulin cause that? By changing the communication that flows between cells.

One of the great insights the authors of this book make clear is cells talk to each other. In this way, they maintain order throughout the system. Health is a consequence of that order. When cellular communication occurs normally, the body functions as it was designed to—flawlessly.

One of the key regulators of cellular communication is insulin. In decades past, we doctors used to think that this hormone's sole job was to regulate the flow of energy into cells. And while this is, in fact, one of insulin's principle functions, we now know that it does a great deal more than simply act as a gatekeeper for energy. Insulin, it turns out, dramatically affects the flow of information that takes place within cells as well as between them, and thus regulates how cells behave. When insulin levels are healthy and balanced, cells function with awesome precision. The consequence for each of us is good health. But when insulin levels become elevated, and remain high over time, cellular communication breaks down. Cells behave in strange and disorderly ways, thus forming the basis for the multiple epidemics we see today.

The good news is that all of us can control our insulin levels by virtue of the nutrients we consume, and the amount of physical activity in which we engage each day. That means that we can, to a great extent, control how our cells function and, by extension, determine for ourselves whether or not we experience good health.

As I frequently tell my patients, as well as the people who listen to me on Oprah Winfrey's television show, medicine can do a great deal to help you defeat disease and restore your health. But the truth is, you can do more than we doctors can.

Peter Kash, Jay Lombard, and Tom Monte's book shows how you can protect yourself from serious illness, and, in many cases, restore your health if you are already ill. By controlling the foods you eat, the nutrient levels in your body, and the amount of exercise you engage in, you can regulate this essential hormone, and in the process give yourself the gift of good health.

—Mehmet Oz, M.D.

· 1 ·

Insulin: The Key
to Health and Illness

Scientists have long dreamed of the day when they would discover that single agent within the human body that causes most of the illnesses that afflict and kill us. With such knowledge, we could transform the source of disease, restore the body's biochemical balance, and thus prevent most cancers, heart disease, diabetes, and overweight—we might even prevent serious degenerative brain disorders, such as Alzheimer's and Parkinson's diseases, as well as conditions that afflict children, including attention deficit hyperactivity disorder (ADHD). Such knowledge could one day form the basis for effective treatments for these conditions, as well.

That remarkable discovery already has been made. Not only have we identified the underlying source of most serious illnesses, but we are learning how to manipulate it successfully to prevent and treat many of the diseases we just named. That singular, pivotal factor, which is both the source of, and the answer to, the vast majority of today's disorders, is insulin, the hormone produced by the pancreas that allows blood sugar, also known as glucose, to enter cells.

Most people know that insulin is directly involved in the creation of diabetes, an illness that now afflicts some twenty million Americans, including an ever-growing number of children and young adults. But the ill effects of insulin go far beyond diabetes. Insulin, scientists have found, is one of the body's master chemicals, regulating an enormous number of other biological functions downstream.

When maintained at balanced levels, insulin insures the steady flow of energy to your cells. It helps create a healthy body weight, supports the health of your heart and circulatory system, and protects you from many common cancers. It also maintains your emotional health and the clarity of your mind and memory.

But when it is elevated, and remains chronically high, insulin can act like a diabolical computer programmer, rewriting your cellular command codes and wreaking havoc throughout the body. Far from being just a catalyst for diabetes, elevated insulin plays a central role in virtually every major illness we face today, including overweight, obesity, heart disease, cancer, and Alzheimer's disease. It is also central to the creation of attention deficit hyperactivity disorder, mood imbalances, and mental illness. Not surprisingly, it helps determine how long we live.

This simple hormone has such a widespread effect on health because every biological act requires energy. Insulin is needed if cells are to use that energy, which means insulin is involved in all human functions. The sheer ubiquity of the hormone gives it entrée into virtually every nook and cranny, every cell, organ, and system of your body. Consequently, insulin can be a help or a hindrance in everything the body does.

To a great extent, we can control our insulin levels by virtue of the kinds of foods we eat, the quantity of calories we consume, how much we exercise, and how well we cope with stress.

Processed foods, such as bagels, muffins, pastries, candy, and soda, for example, are all rich in calories. They are also packed with the kinds of simple carbohydrates—otherwise known as simple sugars—that drive insulin levels through the roof. Foods high in fat are also rich in calories, and can also contribute to high insulin levels. By keeping insulin levels elevated, these foods contribute to all the degenerative illnesses that afflict and kill most of us today.

On the other hand, unprocessed foods—cooked whole grains, fresh vegetables, beans, and fruit—and many low-fat animal products are low in calories and keep insulin levels down. This is one of the major reasons why these foods are associated with good health and longer life.

Exercise, even a simple walk around the block, lowers insulin levels and makes cells more sensitive to the insulin that's in the blood. That means that the body utilizes insulin more efficiently—in other words, a little goes a long way.

In addition, stress drives up insulin levels, and chronic stress keeps insulin levels high. This is one of the ways stress contributes to a variety of major illnesses and premature death: It drives insulin levels up.

Only recently did researchers become aware of insulin's central role in health. But already, scientists have developed new pharmaceutical agents that protect us against the destructive chemical cascade that insulin triggers within our cells. New drugs and dietary approaches that utilize this new understanding are available to address everything from overweight and heart disease, to various kinds of cancers.

In fact, the understanding of insulin's role in health and illness is revolutionizing health care. New forms of treatment offer hope to even those of us who already suffer from one of the many diseases that have been brought about by chronically high insulin levels.

A UNIFIED THEORY

When we, the authors of this book, began our very different paths into the worlds of health and health care, most illnesses were seen as the consequence of a pathogen such as a bacterium or virus, or the result of a general destruction of the body, usually caused by an array of environmental poisons. No common cause of disease could be identified, nor was there any unified field theory concerning health and illness. Rather, scientists and doctors saw various disease states as individual conditions, most of which were unrelated to each other.

Indeed, as a medical doctor and chief of neurology at Bronx-Lebanon Hospital, in New York City, Jay Lombard, treated patients every day from exactly this standard medical paradigm. Major illnesses have long been seen as distinct entities that require individualized forms of treatment. There were few if any common factors that, if manipulated, could help the person with, say, breast cancer as much as it could the person with heart disease. At least that has been the thinking up till recently.

Peter Kash is a venture capitalist who specializes in creating biopharmaceutical companies that offer new and effective medical therapies, especially against cancer and other forms of degenerative illness. Each new treatment that Peter supported for one disease like prostate cancer was, in fact, distinctly different from the drugs he helped fund to treat diabetes, or attention deficit hyperactivity disorder, or Alzheimer's disease.

Under the old medical model, doctors and pharmaceutical companies were restricted to treating the symptoms of disease, rather than the underlying cause of it. In fact, there were too many causes for scientists to identify and treat any single underlying root. Not only has our lack of understanding of the root causes of illness limited our ability to offer more effective treatments, but it has also kept us from creating new programs for prevention.

One of the most baffling mysteries of disease is how it arises. What conditions allow a tiny and dangerous flame within us to become a blazing threat to our lives? Is it true that the body, for no discernible reason, suddenly breaks down, malfunctions, and sets loose a disease process? Or is it possible that an array of poisons—many of which we control—combine to target a single weak link within us, a link that, when it breaks down, sets off a terrible chain reaction?

For many millions of us today, that is precisely what happens. That vulnerable link within us is insulin.

It was Dr. Lombard's careful reading of the medical literature that first alerted us to insulin's biochemical links to illnesses other than diabetes. What Dr. Lombard did, in effect, was back up and see the big picture. Groups of researchers have been working for some time on insulin's relationship to specific illnesses—cancer, for example, or heart disease. Each of these groups focused on its own area of expertise. Few researchers stood back and realized that insulin was a common trigger in virtually all serious illnesses. After Dr. Lombard's realization, he and Mr. Kash both began looking at the scientific literature, which showed that the effects of insulin imbalances on the body are virtually universal.

Insulin is a kind of computer programmer, determining where signals are sent within the human body. Depending on the skill of that programmer, we can experience good health, vitality, and optimal weight and brain function, or we can suffer increasing weight, internal chaos, an endless variety of negative symptom states, and eventually a serious illness.

The growing awareness of insulin's pivotal role in health is changing the way we treat disease, and bringing forth a new model for health and illness. In fact, it is even changing the way we see the human body.

Scientists now realize that the human body is literally the most elaborate and complex array of information highways ever conceived of. Your body can be seen as a living, breathing supercomputer. The health of that supercomputer depends on its ability to send life-sustaining information from one cell to another. That same information must also be transferred to specific sites within cells, so that cells function properly. Illness arises when disruptive or chaotic commands are sent to cells, which in turn cause them to behave in self-destructive ways. In short, proper functioning of the body depends on the information being sent throughout the system.

All of which brings us back to that little pancreatic hormone that we know as insulin. This chemical substance is, in fact, one of the body's central messengers, telling cells to perform an array of essential tasks.

The first job it tells cells to do is to absorb blood sugar (glucose), which is the body's primary fuel. Cells need glucose to perform their tasks, but more fundamentally, they need it to survive. Without blood sugar, cells die.

At the same time, insulin also triggers a series of internal signals within the cells, some of which eventually make their way to your genes, which in turn direct the cell to perform some kind of task. All well and good. But when insulin levels become elevated—and remain high—bad signals get passed to cells and sometimes to your genetic coding, which, once disrupted, can cause any number of serious diseases. The important point to remember for now is that insulin regulates much of the information that gets inside your cells.

Illnesses such as overweight, breast and prostate cancer, diabetes, heart disease, and brain and nervous system disorders appear to be quite different from each other. But let us imagine that each of these illnesses is a specific byproduct, a kind of terrible fruit that springs from the same tree. That tree is called *insulin resistance*.

HOW INSULIN RESISTANCE ARISES

Like any machine, the body needs only a limited amount of fuel to run properly. But unlike other machines, excess fuel is dangerous to the human body. As sugar levels rise, the body experiences dramatic shifts in fluid levels, increasing the risk of edema throughout the system, including in the brain. Brain swelling can lead to coma and death. At the same time, elevations in blood sugar can cause electrolyte levels to drop. Electrolytes are the minerals in cells that facilitate the flow of electrical signals throughout the system. As electrolyte levels fall, organs begin to malfunction. Among the most vulnerable is the heart, which can go into arrhythmia and heart failure.

In order to avoid that fate, the body employs a number of strategies, one of which is to burn off as much of the excess fuel as it can. When there is too much sugar in your blood, the brain signals the pancreas to produce more insulin, and insulin forces the excess sugar into cells so that it can be burned as energy. Unfortunately if the cells are already filled to capacity with sugar and they don't want any more fuel, they close their doors and become "resistant" to the additional glucose. The excess blood sugar remains but if it's not taken care of, you will die. So, doing what it must, the body produces even more insulin, which can then force the excess sugar into cells. Additional insulin can overcome the cell's resistance, but as more and more sugar floods the blood stream, cells put up even more resistance. This resistance is overcome when the pancreas is signaled to make even more insulin.

When cells are persistently overstimulated by a particular signal—in this case, insulin—they eventually become inured, or insensitive, to that signal. In effect, they become resistant to it. High levels of glucose and insulin in the blood cause the insulin receptors on cells to become insensitive to insulin signaling. That's especially the case when the cell is already filled to capacity with glucose.

Insulin resistance is essentially a condition in which cells are rejecting the fuel they need to not only function efficiently but to live. Without fuel, cells die, so the organs they compose (heart, kidneys, etc.) become heavily scarred and lose their functional capacities.

As cells turn glucose and insulin away, more of both fill the blood stream. The body is forced to convert the excess glucose into fat, which accumulates in the blood and throughout our bodies. Some of that fat is stored on the waistline, buttocks, thighs, shoulders, and back, causing excess weight gain. Even more fat forms around the heart and other organs, forcing them to have to work harder to get the same job done. Meanwhile, globules of fat infiltrate the blood, cutting off oxygen supply to cells and organs and causing them to suffocate. Without oxygen, and because of reduced circulation, some tissues die, while others become gangrenous and must be amputated. Atherosclerosis arises in arteries throughout the body, including those leading to the heart. Other organs become deprived of blood and oxygen as well, leading to blindness, kidney disease, impotence, and even gangrene.

As we will see in chapter 5, insulin resistance leads to higher levels of inflammation, which further exacerbates the entire disease process.

The accumulating fat on your body, coupled with the high insulin levels, cause your fatty tissues to produce chemicals that either trigger, or promote, cancerous cells and tissues in the breast, prostate, colon, and lung, among other locations. High levels of insulin can also change the way the cells in your brain function, altering brain chemistry and creating biochemical changes that lead to memory loss and dementia. Elevated insulin levels create a domino effect that can lead to devastating damage in many systems and organs in the body.

· · ·

Now that insulin has been revealed as the basis for so many health problems, scientists are investigating how they can intercept the bad commands initiated by insulin and insert new information that would cause the cell to react properly. In fact, as we will show throughout this book, new drugs are now being developed to do exactly that. And such drug development is being done in virtually every area of health care, from the treatment of overweight and heart disease to cancer and Alzheimer's.

Among the more exciting possibilities is that scientists and doctors will soon be able to tailor diets and lifestyles to fit specific gene profiles and illnesses that the patient faces. Medical doctors will soon be able to prescribe specific foods, exercise habits, changes in lifestyle, and pharmaceutical remedies tailored precisely for your physical makeup and condition.

In the meantime, there is much each of us can do to protect ourselves and those we love, even without our doctor's help.

As Oprah Winfrey's medical guru and renowned Columbia University Medical Center heart surgeon Dr. Mehmet Oz, has said, "We can do a lot for the patient, but the patient can do so much more for himself or herself."

Controlling insulin is important not only from the standpoint of prevention, but also for those who are already ill. Lowering insulin levels can have a dramatic and restorative effect on health, and in many cases, help people overcome life-threatening illnesses. We can prevent disease, restore our health, and also bring our health care costs down.

But in order to do all of that, we must better understand the enormous role insulin plays in the complex and delicate communication that takes place within our bodies.

· 2 ·

Cells Communicate for Health—
If Insulin Allows

It's a little hard for us to imagine that the chemicals passed between cells—including hormones such as insulin—are actually loaded with information, but that's precisely the case. Molecular compounds such as insulin tell cells to behave in distinct ways. These chemicals direct the immune system to produce more natural killer cells, for example, or to attack a virus or bacteria within the system. They regulate the acid-alkaline balance, otherwise known as the blood's pH. They tell cells to reproduce, or to remain stable, or even to self-destruct. In fact, scientists have recently learned that health is the consequence of life-sustaining information being passed between cells and then to specific targets within them. When that information reaches its intended destination, your cells, organs, and, indeed, your entire body functions with beautiful and miraculous efficiency.

On the other hand, many types of chronic illnesses are the

consequence of misinformation passing from malfunctioning cells to healthy cells, which in turn causes cells, organs, and systems to malfunction. Like a virus within your computer, aberrant commands can alter the function of your cells, as well as your body's most elemental form of intelligence—your genes—and thus lead to illness and death.

The process by which cells communicate with each other is called *signal transduction*, and our understanding of this cellular communication is revolutionizing science.

In order to facilitate communication, groups of cells are arranged in neighborhoods, which are closely monitored and coordinated so that individual cells do not act arbitrarily or without regard to the overall good of the system. Within those neighborhoods, signals are passed back and forth between cells, instructing some cells to multiply, others to remain quiescent, and still others to actually commit suicide.

Once a cell receives a signal from one of its neighbors, new signals are triggered inside the cell. Now a new set of messenger proteins race along pathways within the cell, pathways that are more complex than any subway system ever conceived of by human imagination. Eventually, the right messenger protein makes its way to specific targets within the cell, but not before the cell has made a set of highly complex decisions about what signals to send, and what genes to stimulate in order produce just the right action.

If all of this sounds just a bit mind-boggling, well, you are glimpsing the dilemma scientists themselves are struggling with every day. Researchers say that it may take many decades before they figure out the vast cellular "wiring diagram" that exists in all of us.

In order to better understand the process, and how insulin can affect it, we ventured to the laboratory of one of the world's leading specialists in the field of cellular communication, or what is now referred to as *signal transduction*.

CELL COMMUNICATION

The Princeton University campus is dominated by gray collegiate Gothic architecture, with its spires, castle turrets, and gargoyles. These neo-Oxford influences are balanced by many dozens of modern buildings, all of which are low and accessible. The other dominant features of the campus are its trees—they're everywhere—and the many grassy squares and cozy niches that seem to beckon couples and cohorts to their benches for intimate conversation. To walk across the campus is to be enveloped in an atmosphere that seems infused with the presence of great thinkers and artists who graced these lawns and buildings—Einstein, Feynman, Toni Morrison, Anthony Burgess, just to name a few.

In one of the campus's more modern structures, the Lewis Thomas Laboratory, you will find one of the world's leading scientists of our day, Jim Broach, PhD, a pioneer in the field of signal transduction, or the study of how cells pass information within and between themselves.

Broach, in his midfifties, is gray haired and fit. He has a square jaw of a former athlete and small, round eyes that blink frequently when he's trying to formulate his carefully constructed answers. His official title at Princeton is professor of molecular biology and associate director of the Lewis-Sigler Institute for Integrative

Genomics, a title that sums up the range of his expertise on the subjects of cell function and gene theory. When Dr. Broach described, at least in part, the latest scientific understanding of how cells function and maintain health, he began with a startling revelation.

"Cells think," he says matter-of-factly. "They have intelligence. The cell has to take information from multiple inputs and bring them together and balance them out and then decide on a behavior that is informed by all of those different inputs. That processing of information from multiple inputs and then giving an appropriate and coherent response is what I think of as cells thinking."

Though Broach's work occurs primarily in single-cell yeast, much of what he is discovering is also being found in mammalian cells, including our own. "I was surprised to find that one of my colleagues—a colleague with whom I had not discussed this—uses exactly the same term: that cells think. We have found this in yeast cells, and he's found it in mammalian cells. But it's exactly the same idea."

Right now, for example, your cells are being bombarded by an enormous volume of information that is flowing in your blood stream. They are evaluating, for example, the availability of oxygen, protein, and nutrition; the presence of disease-causing agents; the blood's temperature; the availability of fuel; and the level of insulin present in the blood. Elsewhere in the body, nerve cells are sensing your clothing, your weight on the chair, the temperature in the room you are sitting in, and the availability of oxygen in that room. Cells in your eyes are converting the light images that emerge from this page into nerve impulses that are sent on to your brain, enabling you to read. In each instance, your cells are making decisions about how to respond to the stimuli with which they are being bombarded.

"The decisions a cell makes determine whether you maintain health or whether your body is thrown off homeostasis, such as when you suffer from a disease such as diabetes," says Dr. Broach.

Understanding that cells think is a recent insight for scientists. Not only do cells weigh information and give an intelligent response, but they also communicate that response within the cell—that is, to targets within the cell, such as specific genes—and then to other cells within the larger organism.

But the challenge to communicate effectively within organs composed of millions of cells, and to the body at large, composed of trillions, is beyond comprehension. Understanding how this remarkable feat is accomplished is the task Dr. Broach and other scientists like him have set for themselves.

CELL COMMUNICATION IS HOW THE BODY IS SCULPTED TO PERFECTION

Like all multicellular animals, each of us developed from a single cell that doubled, and then kept doubling. At five days after conception, we were little more than a tiny embryonic dot, no bigger than the period at the end of this sentence. From that doubling of cells came a fully formed human being. Such a feat was made possible, in part, by the ability of our cells to specialize, or differentiate, into some 200 different varieties. Hundreds of millions of cells took on specialized abilities to form the brain, others the heart, and still others the digestive tract, reproductive organs, arms and hands, legs and feet. Like good baseball players, our cells took up their positions and matured, each contributing to the body parts, organs, etc. that come together to create a human being.

Of course, that was just the beginning. The estimated three trillion cells that make up your body must cooperate with each other if the human body is to form and health is to be maintained. In order for this to happen, cells must communicate. Groups of cells begin to work in close contact with each other, like neighborhoods, with each community exerting a kind of social control over its members. No cell, for example, is allowed to multiply without express instructions from its neighbors. Those same neighbors also tell the cell when to stop multiplying and enter a more quiet or restful phase. The same is true for many other cellular functions. Every time a cell starts to act independently, the entire organism is in jeopardy.

Cancer is but one example. Essentially, cancer is a disease characterized by cells that mutate—or undergo genetic changes—that cause them to reproduce continually. Neighboring cells command malignant cells to shut down and even to self-destruct. Unfortunately, the cancer cells become disassociated from the signals from other cells. Instead of shutting down, the cancer cells continue to replicate without regard to the health of the overall organism. The result is the overpopulation of certain types of cells that use up vital resources, yet perform not vital tasks. They are autonomous tumors, gobbling up the blood and oxygen of the body, while ignoring the signals from neighboring cells to cease growing. Cancer is a disease that arises when cell communication breaks down.

Cells communicate with each other, says Dr. Broach, by passing messages back and forth in the form of protein molecules, also known as *cytokines*. Each cytokine gives a specific set of orders to neighboring cells, or sometimes to those at a distance. Cells can receive messages because they are equipped with a specialized receptor—think of it as the baseball player's glove—which is itself composed of protein.

Though proteins are the primary source of communication between cells, other specialized cells can create different types of signals. Endocrine cells, for example, create and send hormones such as insulin, testosterone, and estrogen that travel through the bloodstream and can target distant cells. Nerve cells known as neurons create chemicals known as *neurotransmitters* that give rise to moods and mental states such as optimism or depression, relaxation or alertness. Neurons also rely on electrical signals that fire within and between the nerve cells.

Once a cell receives a hormone, cytokine, or neurotransmitter, it initiates another series of internal messengers within itself. These messengers relay information to different stops on pathways toward an ultimate goal—oftentimes a specific gene, or set of genes, within the cell's headquarters, or nucleus.

Within cells, the messenger proteins that travel along the cell's inner pathways are enzymes known as *kinases*. So far, scientists have identified as many as 500 kinases. These proteins act as catalysts, either turning on a cell function, or turning it off. Not only are there hundreds of kinases, but they often undergo changes that further refine and alter their commands. One of the primary ways kinases are altered is through a process called *phosphorylation* that chemically and electrically alters the kinase signal so that it can activate or inhibit a specific cellular activity.

The process is not unlike a basic ground ball to third base.

Once the original signaling molecule is caught, it is then fired to, say, second base, which passes it on to first, and then home. In the cell, these pathways are almost infinitely complex, with many different stops along the way.

The human body is ablaze with crisscrossing lines of information, flowing within cells and between them, at breathtaking speeds. The transfer of information from the tip of your toe to your brain can occur at speeds of 100 meters per second. This speed of information is one of the reasons why we can recognize an oncoming car barreling down the street, assess the danger, and quickly move out of its way—all of which occurs in a matter of milliseconds. Now imagine those same speeds occurring within a microscopic-size cell and you begin to get an idea of the rate of difficulty involved in mapping the inner pathways of cells.

Not only do scientists have to contend with the speed with which information flows, but also the body's vastly complex inner circuitry, now referred to as the "wiring diagram." At one point in our discussion with Dr. Broach, he took out a scientific journal that contained a drawing of only some of the pathways that are known within a single cell. Those pathways were so complex that they resembled the London subway system—only *doubled*.

To make matters even more challenging—and delicate—a cell receives not just one signal at a time, but many all at once. If we use our baseball analogy again, we might say that it isn't just one ground ball to third base, but literally dozens of ground balls being fired to dozens of bases, all at the same time—and all the players getting it right!

"For many years," says Dr. Broach, "we as biologists have been studying how any one signal impinges on and changes the behavior of a cell. And we have learned that different signals change the cell in different ways. Some signals tell the cell to grow, some tell it to stop growing. What we are learning now is that the cell doesn't get a single signal, but multiple signals at the same time, and it has to decide what is the appropriate response at that moment."

Which brings us to an even deeper mystery that, as yet, cannot be fully explained. Some form of intelligence, buried deeply within cells, is organizing each cell's response to the incoming information. That intelligence is the true source of your physical, emotional, and intellectual health.

Though we don't fully understand this organizing intelligence, scientists do know at least one place from which it functions: a tiny array of proteins known as *transcription factors*. These transcription factors regulate the function of genes, in effect turning specific genes on and off.

Transcription factors are located around our DNA and are constantly issuing commands to our genes. We have between 20,000 and 30,000 genes, which contain our biological inheritance. Transcription factors are signaling those genes to produce specific proteins, such as muscle protein, or immune proteins that destroy disease and maintain health.

Unlike a computer, which does little more than accept incoming data, transcription factors receive the information and then make precise decisions in order to produce the best and most appropriate adaptation to the existing events. Transcription factors, for example, will determine which signals to send within the cell, which pathways those signals will travel upon, and which genes will be expressed or shut down. It does this by sending kinases along specific pathways to targeted genes. Transcription factors also order the cell to send out signals to other cells to form a coordinated response in the body.

The role of transcription factors and their effect on our genes disabuses us of one of the more popular cultural beliefs, which is that genes are the ultimate arbiters of our fate. In reality, genes are more like instruments in a grand symphony, each one waiting for the moment when the maestro will point the baton and call forth its music. Genes determine a great deal of our underlying nature, but transcription factors—the cellular maestros—are triggering our genes or keeping them quiet. The delicate virtuosity with which our cells are able to express each relevant gene—and do it at just the right moment—determines our health, and indeed our fate.

"Think of transcription factors as a kind of aristocracy within the cell," Dr. Broach says. "Not only are they taking in and balancing lots of information, and making a decision about that information, but they are also regulating a large number of genes," sometimes as many as fifty genes or more. Once the transcription factor makes its decision, it sends a kinase to trigger a particular gene or group of genes.

For example, transcription factors trigger just such a sequence when you experience pain. Following a bodily injury, there is an increase in the activity of certain transcription factors located in the spinal cord and sensory neurons. These transcription factors stimulate the production of specific molecules that increase inflammatory proteins and generate pain signaling to the brain. Your body knows that it has been injured because transcription factors are passing along that information to your brain.

HELPING OR HINDERING COMMUNICATION— AND THE CELL'S GREAT DECISIONS

Insulin plays a critical role in the vast majority of cell signaling. When balanced, insulin facilitates the smooth flow of information and overall health. But when insulin becomes chronically elevated, or when insulin resistance sets in, breakdowns occur throughout the body and its systems.

For example, insulin, to a great extent, determines your body weight and, more specifically, how much fatty tissue your body carries around. The more insulin there is in your blood, the fatter you become. The fatter you are, the larger your fat cells become. The bigger your fat cells the more likely it is that something will go wrong.

Fat cells are highly active tissues, producing a variety of chemicals, most of which are detrimental to health. Among the more damaging of those chemicals are cytokines that promote inflammation throughout the body, thus increasing your chances of getting heart disease, high blood pressure, diabetes, cancer, arthritis, asthma, and other inflammatory illnesses. These poisonous cytokines also stimulate increased cell division and cancer.

In an insulin-resistant environment, cells grow new and different types of receptors that make them highly sensitive to insulin in the bloodstream. In a high-insulin environment, those receptors are constantly being stimulated, signaling cells to divide, multiply, and proliferate, often without regard for their neighbors or for the good of the body as a whole, thus dramatically increasing the likelihood of developing some form of cancer.

Certain types of cancers, such as colon cancer, display excessive amounts of receptors for insulin, a fact that has caused scientists to theorize that cancer cells depend upon an increase in insulin signaling to promote tumor growth. Many researchers now believe that insulin feeds cancer cells.

In addition to producing poisonous cytokines, fatty tissues also pump out great volumes of sex hormones such as estrogen, which can also serve as cancer promoters. Estrogen is not cancer-causing of itself, but metabolites of estrogen—the byproducts of estrogen utilization by the body—can stimulate the growth of cancer.

As if all of this were not enough, insulin resistance can also change the way kinases behave, which in turn can damage the cell's DNA, thus preventing cells from responding to neighboring cells commands. One of the great decisions cellular neighborhoods have to make is to order a cell, or groups of cells, to commit what biologists refer to as *apoptosis*, or "programmed cell death." Every cell is equipped with a self-destruct sequence, which is an essential program that enables the body to rid itself of potentially harmful cells. In a system that is continually striving for homeostasis, there is no room for unneeded cells. The body must eliminate cells that do not mature or differentiate, or do not perform any needed task, but instead take up space and consume needed resources. These vagrant cells also pose a threat to the system, because they can become cancerous. Indeed, cancer is an ever-growing group of cells that do not differentiate, but instead gobble up resources and turn healthy organs into nonfunctioning masses of tissue.

Insulin resistance often leads to the increased production of growth hormone, which in turn corrodes the gene inside of cells that is responsible for triggering apoptosis. Thus, when the neighborhood cells recognize that one of their cohort is growing out of control, they tell the renegade cell or cells to initiate programmed cell death. But thanks to the effects of the growth hormone, the mutant cells have broken free from the neighborhood constraints and can act independently, without regard for the overall organism.

The body relies on apoptosis in order to maintain the overall integrity and function of organs. Indeed, during fetal development, when organs are rapidly being formed, the body uses apoptosis to "sculpt" organs, cleaving away unneeded tissue. This is especially important in the brain, with its highly complex regions and geography—the cerebrum, cerebellum, limbic system, and hypothalamus, for example. When the fetus is growing inside the mother's womb, cells are multiplying within the blink of an eye. Apoptosis helps to keep each of the brain's regions in the right proportion to each other. It also helps to maintain the brain's structural integrity throughout life, as it does for every other organ in the body (about which, much more in chapter 9).

Unfortunately, high insulin levels may interfere with this process. New research is now showing that chronically high insulin during fetal development interferes with apoptosis and thus allows parts of the brain to grow disproportionately large. Some researchers now believe that this failure of apoptosis may play a role in the onset of autism.

As you can easily see, getting just the right amount of apoptosis—without destroying essential organs—is a delicate feat, one that depends on precise communication between and within cells.

Here again, insulin can be a facilitator of that communication, or a hindrance.

Just as high insulin and insulin resistance can block apoptosis from occurring in some cells, it can also trigger unwanted programmed cell death in others. Much to our horror, insulin resistance in the brain can stimulate unwanted apoptosis in neurons, causing whole swaths of brain cells to destroy themselves and thus bring on memory loss, dementia, and Alzheimer's disease. New research is now showing that Alzheimer's may be a form of "diabetes of the brain."

When brain levels of insulin remain high, neurons begin sending out messengers that trigger apoptosis in brain cells. Cells initiate programmed cell death. Many brain functions degrade and vast swaths of memory are lost, forming the basis for Alzheimer's disease. Chronically high insulin can interfere with the balance of neurotransmitters in the brain, thus forming the basis for an array of other mental and emotional imbalances, especially in children. Several recent studies have shown abnormally high levels of insulin-related growth factors in the spinal fluid of children with autism. Researchers point out that a precise balance of these growth factors is essential for normal brain development. However, when insulin-related growth factors become abnormally high, this delicate balance is disturbed, causing certain parts of the brain to become overly developed—the very abnormalities we have seen in children with autism.

Insulin signaling is involved in the multiple epidemics we face today, including overweight, obesity, heart disease, certain cancers, hyperactivity and attention deficit disorders in children, and an explosion of neurological diseases, including Alzheimer's. At face value, all of these illnesses look distinctly different from one another. But as scientists investigate their deeper origins, they are discovering that all illnesses spring from the same underlying source: insulin resistance, the hidden plague that is destroying the lives of both young and old.

· 3 ·

Overweight, Metabolic Syndrome, and Diabetes—All the Consequence of High Insulin

Bill Diamond, married and father of three, was thirty-nine years old and fifty pounds overweight. His cholesterol level was dangerously high at 250 mg/dl (milligrams per deciliter of blood) and his triglycerides (blood fats) were even worse at 270 mg/dl. He had heart disease, high blood pressure, respiratory distress, and gout, a form of arthritis common among those who eat a high-fat, high-protein diet. He also suffered occasional chest pains. Finally, his fasting blood glucose level was 125 mg/dl, which meant that he was borderline diabetic. His doctor had already told him that he was "insulin resistant," meaning that his cells were so stuffed with blood sugar that they were trying to block any more fuel from entering. When cells try to refuse to accept blood sugar (glucose), it means that there will be an overabundance of sugar in the blood, a dangerous condition that can lead to severe edema, brain swelling, diabetic coma, and death.

HEALTHY BLOOD VALUES, BY THE NUMBERS

Blood cholesterol is divided into types, or fractions. Low-density lipoprotein (LDL cholesterol) causes heart disease and is linked to other serious illnesses. High-density lipoprotein (HDL cholesterol) protects the heart and arteries by taking LDL away from arteries and leading it to the liver, where it is neutralized and passed into the intestinal tract for elimination from the body. For this reason, HDL cholesterol is often referred to as the "good" cholesterol.

Total cholesterol is the number indicating the combined values of both HDL and LDL cholesterol.

The National Heart, Lung, and Blood Institute recommends that your LDL cholesterol should be lower than 100 milligrams per deciliter of blood (usually expressed as mg/dl). But many experts would like to see LDL fall into the 80s or even the 70s.

The U.S. Surgeon General recommends that HDL levels be 60 mg/dl or higher.

Ideally, totally cholesterol should fall around 150 mg/dl. Studies indicate that people with a blood cholesterol level at or around 150 mg/dl have extremely low rates of heart disease. Researchers point out that people with cholesterol levels above 180 mg/dl experience a sharp increase in the risk of heart disease and heart attack.

The Surgeon General recommends that triglycerides (blood fats) should be no higher than 150 mg/dl.

Blood glucose levels are measured in three different ways: a fasting test that is taken after a person has abstained from food for at least twelve hours; a two hour–postprandial test, in which a person has abstained from food for at least two hours; and a random test, taken any time without necessarily abstaining from food.

Healthy values for the three tests are as follows:
Fasting glucose test should fall between 70 and 99 mg/dl
Two hour–postprandial test should range between 70 and 145 mg/dl
Random test should range between 70 and 125 mg/dl

A person is considered diabetic when his or her fasting glucose is 126 mg/dl or higher, or his or her two hour–postprandial test is 200 mg/dl or higher.

Bill's body was responding to his insulin resistance by producing even more insulin, which was forcing the glucose into his cells. But that only made the cells more inflamed.

"Bill," his doctor said, "diabetes shortens a person's life by fifteen years on average. I'm giving you all the drugs we have and they're not reversing the condition. If you keep going like this, you're never going to see sixty-five."

There are approximately twenty million diabetics in the United States. The vast majority—more than seventeen million—have what is called type 2 diabetes (formerly referred to as adult-onset), which arises when the body no longer uses insulin properly. The vast majority of these people are insulin resistant. Typical treatment for insulin resistance and type 2 diabetes includes weight loss, changes in diet, and—if these measures fail, which they often do—medication.

Type 1 diabetes (also known as insulin-dependent diabetes) occurs when the pancreas no longer produces insulin. Because insulin is essential for life, these diabetics must take insulin injections in order to survive.

All diabetics, no matter which form they may suffer from, are far more likely than healthy adults to contract an array of terrible side effects, including heart disease, high blood pressure, gangrene, loss of limbs, blindness, impotence, and kidney disease. Diabetes is the number one cause of blindness and loss of limbs in this country.

There are about twenty million more Americans who are prediabetic, meaning that they have high insulin and are overweight, and therefore are at high risk of contracting the illness. Prediabetics also have an increased risk of suffering from the same related disorders that diabetics incur.

Insulin resistance is the foundation for the vast majority of diabetes in the world. And what most Americans do not realize is that they are eating and slouching their way toward this terrible scourge with every meal they eat.

INSULIN RESISTANCE

When you eat a meal, the nutrients in that meal are absorbed by your small intestine and then into your blood stream. Once in your blood, the carbohydrates from your meal are converted into sugar molecules, now called glucose, which is your body's preferred fuel. The fat in your meal becomes fatty acids (triglycerides) in your blood. These triglycerides are stored in your tissues as fat, which is a future source of energy in the event that calorie consumption falls.

Your brain recognizes the arrival of glucose in your system and responds by telling your pancreas to produce insulin. Once secreted, insulin flows to your cells where it binds with and stimulates a specialized insulin receptor on the cell membrane. That, in turn, triggers a kinase cascade inside the cell membrane that allows glucose to enter the cells. Additional kinases are then triggered that carry the glucose to the cell's mitochondria, the nuclear furnace inside your cells that transforms glucose into adenosine triphosphate (ATP), the substance your cells can use as energy.

Like the gas tank and engine in your car, your cells have a limit to how much fuel they can absorb. If you pump too much gas into your car's tank, the gas will overflow onto the ground. While your car is not going to be affected by the attempt to put in more gas than it can handle, that's not the case with your body. Too much glucose in your bloodstream can cause a diabetic coma and death. Consequently, your brain monitors your blood sugar levels very carefully, and will do all it can to bring glucose levels into the normal ranges as quickly as it can.

When we eat a meal that's rich in calories—calories from fat or from carbohydrates—glucose levels rise rapidly in the blood. The brain recognizes this as an emergency situation and immediately sets two strategies in motion in order to save your life. First, it attempts to burn as much of the blood sugar as it can. The only place it can do that is inside your cells. Therefore, the brain signals the pancreas to produce more insulin, which forces the excess glucose into the cells where it will be burned as fuel.

The second strategy is to store as much of the glucose as it can in your muscles, liver, and fatty tissues, known as adipose tissue.

In order to be stored in your liver and muscles, glucose must be converted to a substance called *glycogen*, which is utilized as fuel whenever glucose levels fall. The remaining glucose will be converted to fatty acids, known as triglycerides, and stored as fat.

Too many carbohydrates become fat on your body because they are converted to triglycerides, and then stored on your stomach, buttocks, legs, and other parts of your body as fatty tissue. Elevated blood triglycerides stimulate your liver to produce more cholesterol, which increases your risk of heart attack and stroke.

While these changes are going on in your liver, muscles, and fat tissue, your cells are being force-fed the excess glucose in your blood, a situation they cannot endure for long. When this situation persists, your cells close down their insulin receptors in order to shut off the flow of fuel. When cells stop accepting glucose, they suffer from a condition doctors refer to as insulin resistance.

Insulin resistance causes biochemical changes that form the basis for an array of serious illnesses. Some of the more dangerous changes are:

- Blood cholesterol levels increase dramatically, causing tissues throughout the body to become inflamed and swollen with cholesterol plaques, including the arteries that lead to the heart and brain. Such conditions, of course, form the basis for a heart attack or stroke.
- High levels of inflammation, among other things, cause the tiny nephrons in the kidneys to become blocked with plaque, reducing their ability to filter and cleanse the blood, a function essential to life. Many diabetics require kidney dialysis to remain alive.
- Circulation of blood is reduced throughout the system. Fingers and toes become numb and prone to infection, nerve damage, and even gangrene. Eventually, this can lead to amputation. When blood flow is impeded to the reproductive organs, impotence is common.
- Weight increases rapidly, leading to the production of hormones that promote even greater weight gain and often to various types of cancers, including those of the breast, colon, and prostate.
- Elevated triglycerides, cholesterol, hormones, and weight combine to create what is called *metabolic syndrome*, a prediabetic condition that can lead to high blood pressure, heart disease, stroke, diabetes, disorders of the joints, circulatory problems,

impotence, and certain types of cancers. As we will see in chapter 6, many scientists now believe that breast and prostate cancers may be a direct result—if not a form of—metabolic syndrome.

• Insulin resistance in the brain can cause the signaling within neurons to become disrupted. Brain cells can turn on apoptosis, or programmed cell death, which eventually can lead to Alzheimer's disease.

Insulin resistance can affect every aspect of our biology, for the simple reason that it disrupts the signaling that occurs within cells. Once the signaling is broken down, cells themselves function in aberrant and destructive ways, which of course leads to illness.

Unfortunately, insulin resistance forces the body to produce more and more insulin in order to get the cells to accept the glucose in the blood.

In his book, *How Fat Works* (Harvard University Press, 2006), Phillip A. Wood, MD, PhD, and director of the Division of Genomics at the University of Alabama, describes insulin resistance this way: Dr. Wood points out that the difference between a healthy person and one who is insulin resistant is that a healthy person immediately experiences a drop in blood glucose levels after his or her body produces insulin. The person who is insulin resistant, however, experiences no significant drop in blood sugar levels, even after his or her body produces significant amounts of insulin. In essence, the blood is still flooded with glucose after a meal—a dangerous condition, as we have said. The body can only react to this situation by producing even more insulin, which will force the cells to accept the glucose into the interior of the cell. The increase in insulin will also cause the body to convert the glucose into fat and store it as rapidly as possible.

As Dr. Wood writes in *How Fat Works*, "Insulin resistance is defined as the condition whereby the body's cells require more and more insulin to get the same effect of glucose uptake."

Insulin resistance is the basis for the onset of diabetes, though most people are insulin resistant for a decade or more before they actually contract diabetes. If you sustain insulin resistance—which means high glucose, high triglycerides, and high insulin—for long enough, you may well contract type 2 diabetes.

Type 2 diabetics produce higher-than-normal quantities of insulin, but also require oral medication to stabilize blood sugar. Nevertheless, the pancreas will have to produce more and more insulin in order to keep pace with the high levels of glucose in the bloodstream. Eventually, the pancreas will give out and lose its ability to produce insulin entirely. At that point, insulin injections will be needed in order for the person to go on living. He or she will no longer have type 2 diabetes, but type 1.

FACTORS THAT LEAD TO INSULIN RESISTANCE

Essentially, there are three factors that lead to insulin resistance: the kinds of foods we eat, our exercise habits (or the lack of them), and our genetic makeup. Researchers are quick to point out, however, that even if you are genetically susceptible to insulin resistance and diabetes, you can avoid both disorders by following a healthy lifestyle.

As an example, scientists point to the Pima Indians of Arizona, who have the highest rates of type 2 diabetes and obesity on earth. Yet their genetically similar cousins, the Pimas of northern Mexico, experience extremely low rates of diabetes and obesity, though they too possess the same genetic vulnerability to both disorders. In fact, the two tribes actually originated from the same peoples who migrated from Asia and settled in North America some 30,000 years ago. One part the tribe made their home in Arizona, while the other went to northern Mexico. Researchers who have studied the two tribes closely have shown that their different disease patterns arise from their very different diets and exercise patterns. The Pimas of Arizona eat a diet rich in fat and calories and lead largely sedentary lives. The Pimas of Mexico eat a diet made up largely of whole grains, vegetables, beans, and small quantities of animal protein. They work hard physically and enjoy various kinds of traditional sports.

These two Pima communities reveal what is happening throughout the United States and around the world: People are eating too many calories and engaging in too little exercise. That's a lethal combination.

A CLEAR PERSPECTIVE ON THE CAUSES OF INSULIN RESISTANCE

The Harvard Medical School in Boston is just a few miles from the more well-known, picturesque campus in Cambridge, across the Charles River. They might as well be two different worlds. The ivy-strewn red brick buildings that are the trademark of the Cambridge campus are nowhere to be seen at the medical school. Here the buildings are gray and tan fortresses, intimidating and blatantly heartless. They are short on art and long on message—an imposing one at that. We do serious work here, these buildings seem to say, and when we look at you, we look with a cold eye.

On the eighth floor of the Beth Israel Deaconess Medical Center at Harvard Medical School you will find George Blackburn, MD, PhD, one of the world's leading experts on insulin resistance, cardiovascular disease, and diabetes.

"We were never meant to eat this many calories," he says. "It's too much for the body," says Dr. Blackburn. "If you look back at the wisdom of our ancestors, you will find that they knew that overeating was bad for your health. They knew to eat smaller meals and to chew the food thoroughly. That was just common sense. Today, it seems we've forgotten a lot of that ancient wisdom."

One of the consequences of our amnesia is insulin resistance, says Dr. Blackburn, and all the problems that go with it.

"It all begins with fatty acids," he says. "Circulating fatty acids get into the machinery of the cell and block the kinases within the cell. Basically, overeating saturated fat and calories causes the cell to become disrupted and brings on insulin resistance."

Dr. Blackburn explains that the fat in our diets is converted in the body to triglycerides, which are composed of three fatty acids riding on the back of an alcohol molecule called a *glycerol*. Triglycerides come from two sources: the fat in our foods, and from the excess calories we consume.

There are drugs to lower triglycerides, Dr. Blackburn points out, but they are not going to have the same effect as simply limiting the amount of fat we eat, especially saturated fat and an artificially produced fat called trans fats.

There are four forms of dietary fat: saturated, polyunsaturated, and monounsaturated fats, and trans fats. By far, the most poisonous are saturated and trans fats, both of which are solid at room temperature, thanks to the fact that both are filled to capacity with hydrogen atoms. Both saturated and trans fats raise blood cholesterol levels, especially the bad cholesterol known as low-density lipoproteins (LDL). Saturated fat is found primarily in animal foods, such as red meat, dairy products, eggs, and chicken. Trans fats are made by food manufacturers who harden vegetable oils—liquid at room temperature—by infusing them with hydrogen atoms, and thus turning them into saturated fats.

Saturated fats and trans fats are more likely to promote insulin resistance and other illnesses, including heart disease. One of the ways they do this is by causing the liver to become inflamed, and disrupting signaling within liver cells. The liver plays a central role in insulin resistance, especially when it has been overfed with lots of fatty acids.

Polyunsaturated fats, which come from vegetable and fish oils, are liquid at room temperature. They lower total blood cholesterol and LDL and offer some protection against heart disease. Monounsaturated fats, which come primarily from olive oil and are also liquid at room temperature, have no effect on LDL, but may raise HDL (the good cholesterol), and thus may also offer some protection against heart disease. As we will see shortly, monounsaturated fats also reduce the size of fat cells and promote weight loss.

Consumption of poly- and monounsaturated fats are associated with lower rates of all illnesses, including diabetes. People who follow a Mediterranean diet, for example, have far lower rates of metabolic syndrome, diabetes, heart disease, and many forms of cancer. They tend to eat relatively more olive oil and significantly fewer animal foods and saturated fats. They also eat dramatically lower levels of trans fats, which are found primarily in processed foods. There is good evidence to show that poly- and monounsaturated fats may also reduce inflammation, thus protecting against a number of serious illnesses.

All fats raise triglycerides, however, and fat is the most calorically dense substance in the food supply. A gram of fat provides nine calories, while a gram of protein or carbohydrate contains only four. A calorie is a unit of potential energy found in food. The more calories we consume, the more potential energy our bodies possess. However, the calories that are not burned as fuel are turned into fatty acids in our blood, and thus can disrupt cell signaling and lead to insulin resistance.

By far, the biggest source of calories in our diets is processed foods, and the more processed, the greater the concentration of the calories in the food. Processed foods include rolls, pastries, bread, cookies, muffins, cakes, candy, soda, processed cheeses, and meats such as bologna, sausage, and pepperoni. These foods are extremely dense in calories. In essence, food manufacturers take a great quantity of natural foods such as corn, or wheat, or potatoes, grind them up, dry them out, cook them down, and turn them into a smaller volume of food. Processing causes carbohydrates to become concentrated, which means that processed foods are going to cause weight gain.

In his book *The Pritikin Principle: The Calorie Density Solution*

(Time-Life Books, 2000), Robert Pritikin shows what happens in the process. A pound of corn, for example, provides 390 calories. But a pound of cornflakes provides 1,770 calories. The same thing happens to potatoes, which provide about 490 calories per pound. A pound of potato chips, however, gives us 2,400 calories. Now, the truth is, you probably couldn't eat a pound of potatoes, at least not in a single sitting, because potatoes are loaded with fiber and water, which provide bulk and thus fill you up, but which contain no calories. Yet plenty of people—especially teenagers—can eat a pound of potato chips without blinking an eye.

Natural, unprocessed grains such as brown rice, millet, barley, quinoa, and whole wheat berries are rich in complex carbohydrates, which are slowly absorbed and do not create spikes in insulin levels. The same is true for other plant sources of carbohydrates, such as squash, turnips, broccoli, and other pulpy vegetables. Not only are the carbs in these foods slowly absorbed, but these foods are essentially low in calories. A pound of brown rice—far more than you could eat in a single meal, or even in a single day—has less than 500 calories. A pound of broccoli, again more than you could eat at a single sitting, has about 85 calories.

But process the carbohydrates in, say, whole wheat, and you can produce a pound or more of bread, which contains about 1,200 calories. When you go to a supermarket today and look down the aisles, most of the foods you see are processed, which means most of them will cause weight gain. You can avoid processed foods by switching to a diet that contains more vegetables, fruit, and cooked whole and unprocessed grains. Another way to lower the calorie content of your diet is to avoid sugar-rich soft drinks.

SOFT DRINKS AND SUGAR: DANGEROUS, ESPECIALLY FOR THE YOUNG

It's common for children and teenagers to wash down snacks with soft drinks such as Coca-Cola, Mountain Dew, Dr Pepper, Sprite, and 7UP. These drinks are little more than "liquid candy," says Michael Jacobson, PhD, director of the Center for Science in the Public Interest (CSPI). The average twelve-ounce can of soda contains ten teaspoons of pure sugar (the equivalent of 40 grams), and 160 calories. (The large Coke sold by McDonald's contains 310 calories.) Needless to say, there is no nutritional value in these drinks, which means that the calories are empty.

On average, Americans consume at least two soft drinks per day, or forty-eight gallons of soda pop a year, CSPI reported. According to the *American Journal of Clinical Nutrition*, carbonated soft drinks are the single biggest source of refined sugar in the American diet.

"Teens just about hit their recommended sugar limits from soft drinks alone," says Dr. Jacobson. "With candy, cookies, cake, ice cream, and other sugary foods, most exceed those recommendations by a large margin."

This is the problem facing American youths today: They're consuming sugar, soda, and processed foods throughout every day of their lives. Not only do many schools have vending machines in their hallways that dispense nothing but processed, sugar-rich foods, but at the same time, the school cafeterias serve an abundance of these same fat- and calorie-rich foods at every noonday meal. The average child's social life is built on calorie-rich sweets.

Consider the ever-escalating trend in children's birthday parties: the "goodie bag syndrome." Our kids spend the entire afternoon eating cake, cookies, pizza, soda, ice teas, and candy, and then are sent home with a bag full of treats—the "goodie bag"—for later in the evening. They're mainlining sugar and calories. Parents feel they must ply the kids with sugar if the party is to be successful. In an average grammar school class, there are between twenty and thirty parties throughout the school year. Is it any wonder that so many are overweight and addicted to sugar and processed foods? If this trend continues, it will not take a crystal ball to figure out that our children's future, and the future of our country, is an adulthood dominated by illness.

THE EFFECTS OF WHOLE FOODS VERSUS PROCESSED FOODS ON YOUR GLUCOSE AND INSULIN LEVELS

Processed foods have a very different effect on glucose and insulin levels than unprocessed foods do. In an unprocessed, natural food, such as squash or brown rice, the carbohydrates are bound up in long chains that are woven into the food's fibers. Those carbohydrates must be worked on by the intestine so that they can be freed from the fiber and their long molecular chains. Little by little these carbohydrates are broken free and released into your blood stream, giving you a long-lasting supply of glucose but keeping insulin levels relatively low.

Something very different happens when you eat a processed food. Processing extracts the carbohydrates from their fibrous chains, turning those complex carbs into simple sugars. Once that's done, the sugars are concentrated in much smaller volumes of food. Some of these simple sugars flow into your bloodstream when they are in your mouth, requiring very little energy for your body to process them. Those that do make it to your small intestine require no breakdown of fiber and no real digestion. These too are rapidly absorbed into your bloodstream. Not only are these sugars quickly absorbed, but they arrive in enormous quantities. It's as if your blood is suddenly flooded with simple sugars, which sends your blood sugar and insulin levels skyrocketing. That, of course, propels the body into an emergency situation in which it must lower its glucose levels as quickly as possible.

STORING GLUCOSE

As glucose floods the blood, the body immediately responds with a spike in insulin levels, and cells are force-fed glucose. Meanwhile, the body tries to store quantities of blood sugar, first in the muscles, and then in the liver. The muscles, which are huge repositories for stored fuel, convert as much glucose into glycogen—the stored form of fuel—as they can. The problem is that if you are insulin resistant or diabetic, your muscles are already packed with unused glycogen. In essence, their fuel tanks are full, which means they can no longer accept additional fuel, or glucose, into their cells. Meanwhile, the lack of exercise causes inactive muscle tissue to lose its ability to utilize glucose, as well as convert glucose into glycogen or stored fuel. There's little or no need for stored fuel in muscle tissue that's not burning much fuel to begin with.

In fact, the inability of insulin resistant muscles to transform glucose into glycogen is severe. In a study published in the *Journal of Clinical Investigation* (July 2000), Gerald I. Shulman, MD, PhD, of Howard Hughes Medical Institute at Yale University School of Medicine, reported that insulin-resistant subjects had a 50 percent reduction in glucose metabolism and glycogen storage, when compared to healthy subjects.

In all probability, the reason is simply that the muscles are already chock-full of glycogen, in part because they have not been exercised. In general, people who are insulin resistant or diabetic tend to avoid exercise and instead lead sedentary lives. Muscles need to be exercised in order to burn off or empty their glycogen reserves. Without exercise, muscles remain full of reserve fuel. Like their cell counterparts, they cannot take in any more excess glucose that shows up in the blood. The consequence is that the blood continues to be flooded with glucose, requiring higher levels of insulin, which in turn must be used to force glucose into cells.

In the face of rising glucose levels, the liver transforms blood sugar into fatty acids to be stored in the adipose tissues as additional fat. This process will add weight to your body. You're not only getting fatter, but your blood is still flooded with both glucose and fatty acids.

The excess fat in the adipose tissues is a reservoir for triglycerides. "Fatty acids are quickly stored in the tissues," says Dr. Blackburn, "but they are also released rapidly into the bloodstream, as well. The blood is flooded with harmful fatty acids, which can lead to insulin resistance."

Many of us think of the fatty tissue around our waist, buttocks, and elsewhere as largely inactive matter, but that is far from the case. The cells in adipose tissue produce hormones and messenger proteins (cytokines) that regulate numerous cellular functions. When these messengers are produced in balanced quantities, cell function often remains normal. But in overweight people, adipose tissue can overproduce both, which in turn can disrupt the cellular function and lead to insulin resistance and other disorders. This is one of the reasons why losing weight is often associated with elimination of insulin resistance. Weight loss reduces adipose tissues and brings hormones and cytokines more into balance. But you have to lose the weight first before you experience a reduction in these dangerous cytokines.

It's worth noting that the current diet and levels of overweight among people are unlike anything we as humans have ever experienced in our two million years of evolution. Processed foods, with their enormous number of calories, are a completely modern phenomenon, and it is only in the last forty years that they have begun to dominate the diet. Our bodies were not designed for an overabundance—and overconsumption—of food, especially when it is sustained, day in and day out. What is far more common in human experience are food shortages and famines, for which the body has adapted protective mechanisms.

One of those protective methods is a process called *gluconeogenesis*, which is the ability of the liver to transform amino acids into fuel (glucose). When food supplies drop and glucose levels fall, the liver will first burn its own glycogen reserves. But when they run out, the liver will convert amino acids into glucose, thus keeping the body alive. When the liver is creating "new glucose" (which is what *gluconeogenesis* means), it is burning fatty acids as fuel. When food is found, and glucose levels rise again, the liver shuts off gluconeogenesis and burns glucose again, thus keeping blood levels of glucose normal.

That's how things function in a healthy state. But in an insulin-resistant state, the liver produces more glucose on its own. There's already too much glucose and fatty acids in the blood, and now the liver adding to the burden. This, of course, forces the pancreas to produce even more insulin in order to force glucose into the cells.

Like finely tuned antennae, the insulin receptors on cells are highly sensitive. Inside the receptor, two delicate protein kinases known as IRS-1 and IRS-2 (IRS for *insulin receptor substrate*) await their orders from the insulin. Under healthy conditions, these two molecules, when phosphorylated by insulin, activate a pivotal kinase within the cell known as PI-3 (*phosphatidylinositol-3*). PI-3, in turn, sets off an entire chain reaction downstream that ensures the smooth flow of glucose from the blood to the appropriate sites within the cell. However, when the blood is too rich in triglycerides, IRS-1, IRS-2, and PI-3 are not properly activated, which in turn prevents the normal kinase cascade from being triggered. The result is a malfunctioning cell, insulin resistance, and elevating levels of glucose and fatty acids within the blood.

This breakdown in signal transduction also affects the mitochondria within the cells, especially those in the muscles and liver. In health, the mitochondria burn glucose and fatty acids. But when cell signaling breaks down, the mitochondria furnaces do not burn fat as effectively. That means that the fatty acids build up even more in the blood, and thus contribute to even greater insulin resistance. All of this results in an even greater overabundance of fuel in the bloodstream.

The brain recognizes this as dangerous, of course, and tells the pancreas to produce even more insulin. The pancreas does its best to produce more insulin, but the beta cells eventually wear out and can longer meet the demands. At this point, the pancreas can no longer produce insulin.

RECOVERY

The key to restoring insulin sensitivity is to reduce the fatty acid content of the blood. Three approaches will do exactly that: weight loss, exercise, and a change in diet to include fewer processed foods, less fat, and more vegetables, whole grains, and fruit.

Weight loss alone will restore insulin sensitivity. Weight loss reduces adipose tissues and fat reserves, which in turn reduces the fatty acid content of the blood. It also reduces the stresses placed on cells by cytokines and hormones.

Exercise also restores insulin sensitivity. As Dr. Wood points out, sumo wrestlers are obese, but they are not insulin resistant. Exercise burns blood sugar and thus lowers insulin. It also forces the muscles and liver to burn glycogen and fatty acids, thus emptying the muscles and allowing them to serve as adequate storage tanks for glucose and glycogen when excess calories are consumed. Exercise also makes muscles more energy efficient. Muscle tissue is very active. Even while the body is largely at rest, muscles will burn more glucose than adipose tissue will. As muscles become larger from exercise, they serve as bigger storage tanks for glycogen. They also become more efficient at transforming glucose into glycogen, which means more fatty acids in the blood get safely stored and eventually burned.

Dietary change is also essential. Fewer processed foods means fewer calories, which translates into weight loss and lower glucose, insulin, and triglyceride levels. Unprocessed foods such as vegetables, whole grains, and fruit are lower in calories, which will promote weight loss and balanced glucose and insulin levels. And fiber-rich foods bind with insulin and help eliminate it from the body, thus lowering the overall insulin level.

All of these factors affect health in a multitude of ways, as we will see in the chapters ahead.

Such advice is age-old, says Dr. Blackburn. "Eight hundred years ago, Maimonides, a famous religious teacher and physician, taught not to overeat, and to eat slowly, and do not overeat fat," says Dr. Blackburn. "These ideas are still true today. They're part of our basic human wisdom. They keep us healthy, but we're not following that today and there are many serious consequences."

One of the biggest consequences of insulin imbalance, of course, is overweight, which is one of the greatest threats to health and life that we face today.

· 4 ·

Curing Overweight and Obesity

We read a lot about the numbers of people who are overweight or obese, but very little about how the growing waistline of Americans is changing attitudes and business. The truth is, everybody is adjusting to the expanded girth. And in some cases, it's designed to make us feel better about ourselves, even as we gain more weight. Here are some examples:

We're making clothing bigger, but labeling it smaller sizes. Today's size 10 dress was sold in the 1940s as size 14. Nike's small sports bra used to fit a woman with a 33- to 35-inch bustline. Today, Nike's small bra is designed for a woman with a 35- to 37-inch bust.

Business at plus-size boutiques is booming. Lane Bryant plans to nearly double the number of its stores nationwide over the next five years. Catherine's Plus Sizes is not far behind. The Gap, Limited, and Target are all selling plus sizes to children now.

We're making seats bigger. When the Boston Red Sox renovated Fenway Park, they made the seats four inches wider. They had to, in order to accommodate the average fan. Seattle's Puget Sound ferries had to create more benches and bigger seats for riders. The old seats were too small, so too many people had to stand.

Doctors are now using longer needles to administer vaccines and medicines, and to draw blood. The old standard needles are too short to fully penetrate the thicker layers of fat on the arms of Americans.

We're allowing more weight on aircraft. The Federal Aviation Administration ordered airlines to add another ten pounds per person to approved passenger weights.

Cosmetic surgery is fast replacing dieting. Liposuction is now the most common cosmetic surgical procedure in the country, having increased 118 percent between 1997 and 2001.

More and more of us have given up hope of ever being at a healthy body weight again. Robert Ferrer was one such example.

Robert stood five feet eleven inches tall and weighed 290 pounds. He was morbidly obese, but that was only part of his trouble. His total blood cholesterol level was 280 mg/dl, which meant that he had galloping atherosclerosis in his coronary arteries. He had high blood pressure and painful bouts of claudication—leg pain caused by poor circulation. He was insulin resistant and taking oral medication for diabetes. He regularly suffered from shortness of breath and occasional arrhythmia, especially when he climbed stairs. His feet were so swollen and numb that he constantly feared infection and the loss of one or more of his toes.

Like so many overweight Americans, Robert was a chronic dieter—he'd tried them all—and although he did occasionally lose weight, he regularly gained back the lost pounds shortly after losing them. The problem was that he couldn't stay on a diet; they all represented some form of unendurable hunger to him. If truth be told, he didn't have much hope of ever succeeding on any weight-loss plan until his doctor explained insulin to him.

Robert thought that dieting was all about calories, which is partially true, but there is more to it than that. In simple terms, we gain weight when we eat more calories than we burn; we lose weight when we burn more calories than we eat. But this formula is actually too simplistic to help in creating a practical and effective weight-loss program, especially for overweight people whose diets chronically fail them.

"Before I understood insulin," Robert recalled, "my diets were either austere or loaded with fat. I was either on the high-carbohydrate, low-fat diet, which didn't give me any real pleasure, or I was on the high-protein, low-carb diet, which made me feel physically and mentally terrible. I couldn't win. But when my doctor told me how insulin works, and I started reading about how insulin is related to weight, I began to understand how I could eat a low-calorie diet that allowed me to enjoy foods that made me feel satisfied and full, but at the same time caused me to lose weight. For example, I love pasta with vegetables cooked in olive oil. And I love to sauté my vegetables in olive or sesame oil. A diet based on the principle of low insulin allowed me to eat all of these foods, and lose weight at the same time."

In fourteen months, Robert lost 100 pounds, and he has kept the weight off for more than two years. "I don't believe I will ever be fat again," he said recently. "I know how to keep my weight down now."

Robert is one of the lucky ones, and, unfortunately part of a minority. Most Americans (two-thirds) are overweight, and half of those are obese. What's worse, the number of overweight and obese people is rising with frightening speed. Twenty years ago, only 15 percent of adult Americans were obese. Today, that number has more than doubled to 30.5 percent.

The problems associated with overweight and obesity go beyond the esthetics of physical appearance, though. When you consider the psychological impact of excess weight on children and adults, that alone should warrant a national effort to help people slim down. Children who are overweight are often ostracized and teased. Many grow up seeing themselves as fat, ugly, and unworthy of love—conditions that affect their entire lives. Obese adults are confronted with situations every day in which their size places them in untenable or humiliating circumstances.

Then there are the health effects of overweight and obesity, most of them lethal. Heart disease, high blood pressure, stroke, diabetes, the common cancers, asthma, and gall bladder disease are just some of the problems associated with the disorder. Today, the costs associated with obesity-related illnesses has reached $117 billion. Overweight and obesity are just behind tobacco as today's leading causes of death and disability.

Body Mass Index (BMI)

The Body Mass Index (BMI) chart on the following page will show you whether or not your weight is in the healthy ranges. BMI takes into account both the quantity of fat on your body and your muscle tissue.

Find your height in the left column and read across and find your weight. The BMI for normal weight falls between 18.5 and 25; a person with a BMI of 25 to 29 is considered overweight and someone with a BMI of 30 or above is considered obese. In general, however, obesity is defined as 20 percent above ideal body weight.

BODY MASS INDEX
The number at the top of that column is your BMI. Check the word above your BMI to see whether you are normal weight, overweight, or obese. If you are overweight or obese, talk with your doctor about ways to lose weight to reduce your risk of diabetes or prediabetes.

Health experts are unanimous in their assertion that the underlying cause of overweight and obesity is poor diet and lack of exercise. Children today have more incentives to be sedentary than to be active. Even sports, the staple of after-school activity, have fallen by the wayside. In the late 1960s, 80 percent of children participated in a sport on a daily basis. Today, only 20 percent do. Television, video games, and the Internet keep children sedentary. It's the rare child who goes out after school to play basketball, soccer, tennis, football, or baseball with friends.

And then there is the problem of food. Has any generation of humans ever been more confused about what to eat than our own?

Body Mass Index

	Normal						Overweight					Obese						
BMI	19	20	21	22	23	24	25	26	27	28	29	30	31	32	33	34	35	36
Height (inches)	Body Weight (pounds)																	
58	91	96	100	105	110	115	119	124	129	134	138	143	148	153	158	162	167	172
59	94	99	104	109	114	119	124	128	133	138	143	148	153	158	163	168	173	178
60	97	102	107	112	118	123	128	133	138	143	148	153	158	163	168	174	179	184
61	100	106	111	116	122	127	132	137	143	148	153	158	164	169	174	180	185	190
62	104	109	115	120	126	131	136	142	147	153	158	164	169	175	180	186	191	196
63	107	113	118	124	130	135	141	146	152	158	163	169	175	180	186	191	197	203
64	110	116	122	128	134	140	145	151	157	163	169	174	180	186	192	197	204	209
65	114	120	126	132	138	144	150	156	162	168	174	180	186	192	198	204	210	216
66	118	124	130	136	142	148	155	161	167	173	179	186	192	198	204	210	216	223
67	121	127	134	140	146	153	159	166	172	178	185	191	198	204	211	217	223	230
68	125	131	138	144	151	158	164	171	177	184	190	197	203	210	216	223	230	236
69	128	135	142	149	155	162	169	176	182	189	196	203	209	216	223	230	236	243
70	132	139	146	153	160	167	174	181	188	195	202	209	216	222	229	236	243	250
71	136	143	150	157	165	172	179	186	193	200	208	215	222	229	236	243	250	257
72	140	147	154	162	169	177	184	191	199	206	213	221	228	235	242	250	258	265
73	144	151	159	166	174	182	189	197	204	212	219	227	235	242	250	257	265	272
74	148	155	163	171	179	186	194	202	210	218	225	233	241	249	256	264	272	280
75	152	160	168	176	184	192	200	208	216	224	232	240	248	256	264	272	279	287
76	156	164	172	180	189	197	205	213	221	230	238	246	254	263	271	279	287	295

	Obese			Extreme Obesity														
BMI	37	38	39	40	41	42	43	44	45	46	47	48	49	50	51	52	53	54
Height (inches)	Body Weight (pounds)																	
58	177	181	186	191	196	201	205	210	215	220	224	229	234	239	244	248	253	258
59	183	188	193	198	203	208	212	217	222	227	232	237	242	247	252	257	262	267
60	189	194	199	204	209	215	220	225	230	235	240	245	250	255	261	266	271	276
61	195	201	206	211	217	222	227	232	238	243	248	254	259	264	269	275	280	285
62	202	207	213	218	224	229	235	240	246	251	256	262	267	273	278	284	289	295
63	208	214	220	225	231	237	242	248	254	259	265	270	278	282	287	293	299	304
64	215	221	227	232	238	244	250	256	262	267	273	279	285	291	296	302	308	314
65	222	228	234	240	246	252	258	264	270	276	282	288	294	300	306	312	318	324
66	229	235	241	247	253	260	266	272	278	284	291	297	303	309	315	322	328	334
67	236	242	249	255	261	268	274	280	287	293	299	306	312	319	325	331	338	344
68	243	249	256	262	269	276	282	289	295	302	308	315	322	328	335	341	348	354
69	250	257	263	270	277	284	291	297	304	311	318	324	331	338	345	351	358	365
70	257	264	271	278	285	292	299	306	313	320	327	334	341	348	355	362	369	376
71	265	272	279	286	293	301	308	315	322	329	338	343	351	358	365	372	379	386
72	272	279	287	294	302	309	316	324	331	338	346	353	361	368	375	383	390	397
73	280	288	295	302	310	318	325	333	340	348	355	363	371	378	386	393	401	408
74	287	295	303	311	319	326	334	342	350	358	365	373	381	389	396	404	412	420
75	295	303	311	319	327	335	343	351	359	367	375	383	391	399	407	415	423	431
76	304	312	320	328	336	344	353	361	369	377	385	394	402	410	418	426	435	443

The plethora of food and diet experts—many of whom disagree with each other—only seems to make matters worse. Most Americans have tried and failed on a wide variety of diets. Why are we so clueless on a subject that was second nature to our grandparents and forebears?

THE STATE OF DIETING TODAY

Part of the problem with diets and dieting most certainly rests with the fact that we have so many food choices today. There is more food available to us than at any other time in human existence. Meanwhile, food manufacturers have created thousands of new foods that tantalize the tastebuds but do not contribute to our health. Fast food may be convenient and tasty, but it makes us fat and sick. In the supermarket aisles, we must read labels, understand complicated scientific terms, and try to determine if the foods we purchase will cause disease. Food has become complicated and dangerous, which is why so many of us turn to experts for help.

Although there is no limit to the number of advisors out there, there is a limit to the types of diets that are available. Essentially, two regimens have dominated in the last three decades: the low-fat, high-carbohydrate regimen, and the low-carbohydrate, high-protein diet.

Originally, the high-carbohydrate, low-fat regimen was composed largely of unprocessed foods such as whole grains, fresh vegetables, beans, fruit, and low-fat animal products. All of these plant foods are low in calories and rich in nutrition. They also keep insulin levels relatively low. Not surprisingly, many people lost weight on this approach, and thousands more were able to reverse serious illnesses. But the restrictions of the low-fat, high-carb diet—especially when it comes to healthful fats, such as olive, sesame, and safflower oils—make it unsatisfying for many.

During the late 1980s and 1990s, the high-carb diet went through a strange metamorphosis that was largely unnoticed in the press. Food manufacturers, responding to an enormous trend in the marketplace, began offering carbohydrate-rich foods that were highly processed and loaded with calories. They labeled these foods, "Low-Fat!" or "No-Fat!" but they are nonetheless loaded with calories—rapidly absorbed calories, which means they have a devastating effect on insulin levels, raising them through the roof. Thus, the once healthy low-fat, high-carb diet soon became the high-carb, high-calorie, high-insulin diet, which is one of the primary reasons so many people of all ages are overweight today.

The almost-predictable reaction to the failure of the low-fat diet was the high-protein diet, which is low in carbohydrates but rich in fat. That diet caused some weight loss, but people couldn't stay on it because it had a wide variety of side effects, which for many people included constipation, headaches, bad breath, joint pain, and a constant craving for the body's primary source of fuel, carbohydrates. High-protein diets can also promote bone loss, osteoporosis, and kidney disorders, among other serious conditions.

Protein is converted in the body into acid, which is then eliminated from the blood by the kidneys. Your brain monitors your blood acid (pH) levels very carefully. It is continually attempting to maintain a balanced pH or a slightly alkaline state. When blood acid levels rise too high, the brain signals the bones to release phosphorus and calcium, which naturally alkalize the blood and restore its balanced pH. These minerals neutralize the excess acid, but at a price. The loss of calcium and phosphorus weakens bones. If this bone loss continues, your bones can eventually become porous and osteoporotic. High blood acidity also can weaken and eventually injure the kidneys, which are forced to eliminate as much acid from the blood as possible.

High-protein diets, of course, cause elevations in both protein and acid levels within the blood, which sets off a domino effect that can ultimately result in osteoporosis and kidney disease.

By 2005, both high-carbohydrate and high-protein diets had clearly failed, and the high-protein diet, which boomed during the 1990s, faded quickly. Any weight loss achieved on either one was quickly gained back after people abandoned one or both approaches. At this point, most of us are confused, and a great many are cynical, about the whole subject. Meanwhile, the epidemic of overweight and obesity only gets worse.

This does not mean that weight loss and health promotion cannot be achieved. It only means that the two dominant approaches to this point have been unable to satisfy both our palates and our concerns about weight and health.

It's worth remembering that our ancestors, no matter whether they came from Europe, the Mediterranean region, Africa, or Asia never thought about dieting. Yet most were lean. Even today, many populations, especially those in Asia and in the Mediterranean, are still lean and experience relatively lower rates of the illnesses that we take for granted today.

How is this possible? The answer lies in our understanding of insulin.

HOW INSULIN HELPS TO
DETERMINE OUR WEIGHT

To understand insulin's effect on weight, we only need to think of insulin as a storage hormone. The higher your insulin levels, the more fat you store in your tissues, and the more weight you gain because insulin determines how much fat you burn as fuel.

Right now, as you read this book, your cells are utilizing a fuel mix that is composed of about 50 percent glucose and 50 percent fat. As long as your insulin level remains relatively low, you are burning a mixture of blood sugar and fat. But let's say that you eat a piece of white bread, or a bagel, or a doughnut, or some other food that is rich in processed carbohydrates. Immediately, your blood is flooded with glucose. Your body sees this as an emergency situation and releases an abundance of insulin so that your cells will burn as much excess glucose as possible. In order to enhance glucose burning, your brain instructs your cells to stop burning fat—just burn sugar, and nothing else, it says. This will help to bring down your glucose levels into the safe ranges. Your body does this to keep you from going into a diabetic coma.

As we saw in the last chapter, the body usually cannot burn all the calories that are consumed, especially from processed foods. The excess blood sugar that cannot be burned must instead be converted to triglycerides (fatty acids), and stored in your tissues as fat.

All those excess calories in processed foods are not the only problem, however. Most processed foods also contain fat. So, let's say that rather than snacking on a bagel, which contains virtually no fat, you eat potato chips, which are rich in both processed carbs and fat. The carbohydrates in the potato chips go into the blood stream and become glucose. The fat is also absorbed into your blood. Instantly, your body says, "Shut off fat burning and instead burn as much glucose as possible." At the same time, your body stores the fat from the potato chips in your tissues. In addition, any glucose that cannot be burned is also stored as fat in your tissues. Both the fat and the excess carbs become fat on your belly, buttocks, arms, shoulders, and legs.

Like most processed foods, potato chips are high in calories. A pound of potato chips provides about 2,400 calories. The body needs approximately 10 calories to maintain one pound of body weight. That means that that 2,400 calories supports the weight of a 240-pound person. If you eat a pound of potato chips and you weigh less than 240 pounds, you're gaining weight. If you already weigh 240 pounds, and you eat a pound of chips, you're also gaining weight because you are presumably eating more than just the chips that day. Which is why potato chips, like most processed foods, make us fat.

From an insulin, calorie, and weight-loss standpoint, processed foods are uniformly dangerous. They are concentrated packages of calories that are rapidly absorbed and cause insulin to spike and fat to be stored in the tissues. When fat is added to them, they're even worse.

But here's an interesting fact that most of us don't understand. If you eat a mono- or polyunsaturated fat such as olive oil, or sesame oil, or safflower oil with a low-calorie food such as vegetables, you will actually promote weight loss, for two reasons. First, polyunsaturated fats tend to slow the rate at which carbohydrates are absorbed into the blood stream. When cooked with olive oil, carbs tend to enter the blood stream at a slower pace, which keeps insulin levels relatively low. When insulin levels are low, you keep burning fat that's stored in your tissues. Second, mono- and polyunsaturated fats stimulate your body to release stored fat into your bloodstream and burn it as fuel.

In order to understand how this happens, we must have a better understanding of the fat that we're carrying around on our bodies.

WHAT IS FAT TISSUE?

The fat on our stomachs, buttocks, and elsewhere is known as adipose tissue. The cells that make up adipose tissue, called *adipocytes*, are capable of expanding up to 1,000 times their original size. Fat cells can get fat, which, of course, makes us fat.

The body stores fat as a backup fuel source. In fact, our ability to retain fat on our tissues was a form of adaptation that kept our early ancestors alive. As we will see in greater detail later on, people in ancient times—anywhere from 20,000 to 400,000 years ago— who had relatively more fat on their tissues had a better chance of surviving food shortages, long migrations, and winters than those who were too lean. It seems that survival was not only of the fittest, but also of the fattest.

There are two forms of adipose tissue: one is called *visceral fat*, which surrounds the internal organs, such as the kidneys, liver, spleen, and intestines; the other is called *subcutaneous fat*, and is found mostly around the buttocks and the belly.

Visceral fat is highly volatile and shed relatively easily. A little exercise and a reduction in calorie consumption causes this fat to be mobilized and rapidly burned as fuel. The body sees visceral fat as a ready and quick source of energy whenever it is needed. It's analogous to your basic candy bar. If you're playing basketball, or tennis, or out walking, you'll burn the fuel stored in your muscles. Once that's gone, your body will call to its visceral fat to meet its energy needs.

Subcutaneous fat, on the other hand, is much more intractable and stubborn, in large part because the body regards this form of fat as a long-term fuel supply, especially when food shortages endure. Consequently, the body is much more reluctant to surrender it, because it could be a life-saving form of energy when food is scarce. In the modern life, of course, subcutaneous fat is that last ten pounds that are so difficult to shed.

Men tend to have relatively more visceral fat, while premenopausal women relatively more subcutaneous fat. This makes sense from an evolutionary standpoint. Premenopausal women are capable of giving birth. Nature equipped them with more long-term energy supplies in the event of a pregnancy.

Men, who traditionally did more manual labor, need a ready and accessible supply of energy when glycogen levels fall. Hence, the purpose of visceral fat—the quick-pick-me-up fat that is stored around your organs and deep inside your belly and can be rapidly mobilized and burned when instant energy is needed.

Scientists used to believe that adipose tissue—whether visceral or subcutaneous—was nothing more than a storage depot for energy. They also thought that fat was highly inactive—everyone believed that it remained inactive and waited for the moment when it was needed. But recent discoveries have changed these notions.

Adipose tissue, it turns out, is now recognized as an endocrine organ, meaning an organ that produces hormones. Not only is it highly active, but essential for the healthy functioning of the entire body. Adipocytes produce an array of hormones that act as messengers to the entire system. Among them is *tumor necrosis factor*, which, when produced in excess, can lead to inflammation and heart disease (about which, more in chapter 5). They also produce estrogen, the female sex hormone; and a substance called leptin.

LEPTIN: ONE OF THE KEYS TO UNDERSTANDING WEIGHT AND WEIGHT LOSS

Leptin, from the Greek word *leptos*, which means "thin," regulates appetite and food intake as well as glucose and fat burning. When the body has stored enough energy as fat, adipose tissues increase production of leptin, which sends a signal to an organ in the brain called the hypothalamus. The hypothalamus, in turn, sends out a signal to the brain and stomach to stop eating, lose appetite, and recognize that you are now sated. The hypothalamus also signals muscles throughout the body to start burning excess fat stored in the muscles and other tissues. Scientists have identified a kinase within the hypothalamus called AMPK (AMP-activated protein kinase), which signals the hypothalamus to send out the message to stop eating and start burning fat.

At the same time, the burst of leptin tells skeletal muscles throughout the body—again, by stimulating AMPK—to burn glucose and fat supplies in the muscles. That will lower weight all by itself. When the muscles empty their energy supplies, they become good storage tanks for excess glucose and fat for the next time we eat a processed or high-fat food. When the body can store excess glucose and fat, it does not have such high levels of glucose in the blood, which means that it does not have to produce so much insulin. One of the benefits of low insulin is that the body will keep on burning fat as part of its fuel mix.

Thus, under healthy conditions, leptin lowers your appetite, limits your food intake, and keeps you burning both fat and glucose. Leptin also increases insulin sensitivity, which means you need less insulin to do the same job—another way leptin keeps insulin levels low, and fat burning high.

When scientists first discovered leptin in 1994, they immediately thought that they had found the answer to overweight and obesity. Give people more leptin, they reasoned, and they will immediately eat less and burn more fat. Alas, that was not the case. In fact, leptin levels were already higher in obese individuals, researchers soon discovered. And when obese people were given leptin therapeutically, they did not respond as expected. The hypothalamus—the major site of leptin signaling—failed to react to the increase in leptin signaling. As it turned out, the hypothalamus and muscles in overweight and obese people had become resistant to leptin's instructions. Later studies showed that the gene that, under normal circumstances, would otherwise respond to leptin, failed to react to the leptin signaling. Consequently, the hypothalamus did not send out a message to the body to stop eating and start burning fat.

Laboratory studies found that obese mice have higher than normal leptin levels, but they nonetheless sit under the food hopper and continue to eat. They remain hungry long after their stomachs are full and their bodies require no more energy. People respond in similar ways, later studies discovered. In fact, a study published in the medical journal *Diabetes* (April 2002) reported that obese people have higher than normal leptin levels. The leptin simply fails to do its job.

Interestingly, even in overweight and obese people, leptin works for a time, but its messages are eventually overridden and fail. The disorder that arises when leptin no longer makes us feel full, and fails to stimulate fat burning, is called *leptin resistance*.

A study published in February 2006 in the *Journal of Molecular Endocrinology* reported that leptin resistance arises with the elevation of a specific protein, known as PTP1B, that blocks leptin signaling within the cells of the hypothalamus. What increases this pernicious protein? Saturated fat from red meat and dairy products. Researchers found that as saturated fat intake increases, so too does PTP1B, which in turn makes the hypothalamus and muscle tissue resistant to leptin.

In support of such findings, the *British Journal of Nutrition* (October 2000) reported that diets high in saturated fats stimulate more eating and calorie consumption. Saturated fats make us eat more, in part, because they weaken leptin's impact on our appetite.

On the other hand, vegetable oils—specifically monounsaturated and polyunsaturated fats—restore leptin sensitivity and effectiveness. Numerous studies have shown that fish oils—polyunsaturated omega-3 fat—perform the remarkable feat of restoring leptin sensitivity and insulin sensitivity, and promote fat burning.

In a study published in the *Journal of Lipid Research* (August 1998), laboratory animals were fed three different diets, all of which contained the same amount of calories, but different types of fat. One group of animals ate fish oils, another safflower oil, and the third beef tallow. The first two types of oil, fish and safflower, are both polyunsaturates, while the last one, beef tallow, is a source of saturated fat. The study showed that the animals fed polyunsaturated oils had a 60 percent higher production of leptin, while those fed beef tallow experienced a decrease in leptin.

For anyone who is overweight, diabetic, or insulin resistant, a switch from saturated fat to mono- and polyunsaturated fats is an essential step. You will very likely have more control over your appetite, eat less, feel satisfied, and lose weight faster if you eat moderate amounts of polyunsaturated and monounsaturated fats than if you eat saturated fats from beef and dairy products.

Moreover, whole, unprocessed plant foods are nutrient-rich, low-fat foods. When low-calorie plant foods are combined with moderate amounts of olive, sesame, or safflower oil, as well as with low-calorie animal foods, you arrive at a diet that is both low in calories and highly satisfying. In addition, it will keep insulin levels low, which means you will continue to burn fat.

A "moderate amount" of oil is one tablespoon of olive, sesame, or safflower oil, which contains approximately 250 calories. For people who want to lose weight, that tablespoon can be used several times a week or even daily, depending on how much weight you want to lose, and how fast you want to do it. The oil can be used in cooking, or added raw to vegetables. The Mediterranean diet is just one example of how traditional people—the French, Italians, Greeks, Israelis, and North Africans—use precisely this combination of plant foods, low-fat animal products, and oils to create a diet that is low in calories and rich in nutrition. The Mediterranean diet, as you know, is associated with low rates of all the modern illnesses, including heart disease, the common cancers, diabetes, Alzheimer's, and Parkinson's disease. (The dietary guidelines provided in chapter 12 will help you create your own approach.)

Interestingly, one more substance also increases leptin sensitivity: A substance in red wine known as resveratrol acts as a PTP1B blocker and thus restores leptin sensitivity to the hypothalamus and to muscle tissue. Scientists speculated that resveratrol could be one of the keys to the well-known French paradox—the term frequently used to describe the fact that the French people, who drink substantial amounts of red wine and eat plenty of fatty foods, are nonetheless lean. French have relatively low rates of obesity and overweight, especially when compared to Americans.

EXERCISE

Interestingly, researchers have found that exercise, even a twenty-minute walk per day, causes a very similar effect as leptin on the brain, muscles, appetite, fat burning, and insulin levels. In fact, exercise triggers the same kind of signal transduction as leptin on skeletal muscles. Once we begin walking, AMPK is triggered, signaling muscles to burn fat and glycogen stores. At the same time, exercise increases insulin sensitivity. Both of these alterations in biochemistry results in weight loss and lower insulin levels.

These same effects have been found in people in their sixties. Researchers at Case Western Reserve University School of Medicine in Cleveland, Ohio, examined sixteen obese men, all of them sixty-three years of age or older, who walked on a treadmill and/or rode a cycle machine daily. All of them were insulin resistant at the start of the study. No changes in diet were made, but after twelve weeks of walking or cycling, all had lost weight and had overcome insulin resistance (*Journal of Applied Physiology*, December 22, 2005).

Exercise burns calories, of course, but that is not the primary way it causes weight loss. A three-mile walk or run might only burn 350 calories, and you'd need to do ten such walks in order to lose a single pound of body weight (the equivalent of 3,500 calories). Fortunately, burning calories is only one way exercise contributes to weight loss—and perhaps the least efficient way. Exercise builds muscle mass, which is highly active tissue that is constantly burning higher levels of fat, even when you are not exercising. It also improves the efficiency of muscles, increasing fat burning. When muscles are exercised, their glycogen stores are emptied, freeing them up for taking on excess glucose. This means that when glucose levels become elevated—after eating processed food, for example—the body can place more glucose in the muscle tissue and thus maintain lower insulin levels. With lower insulin, more fat is burned, even while you are resting. All of this contributes to weight loss. And with regular exercise, we can move out of insulin resistance.

Exercise physiologists point out that while a daily thirty-minute exercise routine should be the goal, we can accomplish nearly as much with three ten-minute walks per day. Such a program can be greatly enhanced by engaging in an hour of exercise on the weekends, such as walking, either outside or on a treadmill, or riding an indoor cycle machine, or playing a sport that you enjoy. Such an exercise program can give us all the physiological and health-restoring benefits described here. When these movements are coupled with a low-calorie, high-nutrient, high-satiety diet, even obesity can be overcome.

INFLUENCING THE BRAIN
IN ORDER TO LOSE WEIGHT

Nora Volkow, MD, director of the National Institute of Drug Abuse, has shown that food and illicit drugs share the same reward circuitry in the brain. Both increase the neurotransmitter known as *dopamine*. Dopamine, in turn, triggers the reward centers of the brain, which means that both food and drugs make us feel good. And not surprisingly, both can be addictive.

Researchers hypothesize that low dopamine levels may trigger food cravings, even when one is not otherwise hungry for food. Interestingly, scientists have also found that normal insulin signaling in the brain stimulates the release of dopamine. That means that normal insulin function may result in higher dopamine and more consistent states of well-being—thanks to the well-stimulated reward centers—and lower food cravings. That very sequence could explain why many people are not overcome by food cravings and find it easy to maintain normal body weight.

On the other hand, people with insulin resistance experience a decrease in dopamine signaling, which in turn stimulates food cravings. Eating elevates dopamine and alleviates the food cravings, at least temporarily. But as dopamine falls, cravings rise, even when food consumption is harmful.

Findings like these are behind the search for new ways to elevate dopamine and stimulate the brain's reward centers, without turning to food.

WE ARE DESIGNED TO WANT CALORIES AND FAT

In a very real sense, we are designed to accumulate and conserve calories. Our Paleolithic ancestors experienced extreme fluctuations in their food supply, which meant that whenever a large meal presented itself, they gorged on it. Gorging became an essential survival strategy, says Kerin O'Dea, PhD, in her article "Obesity and Diabetes in the 'Land of Milk and Honey'" (*Diabetes/Metabolism Reviews*, December 1992). Our ancestors never knew for certain when their next meal might come, or if it would be adequate to keep them alive.

Gorging, of course, means taking in as much nutrition and calories as possible in a single meal. Most of the food that was available to our ancestors was plant foods, such as roots, tubers, stems, leafy vegetables, and fruit. We supplemented these foods with wild game, which provided fat, the single greatest source of calories in the food supply. The fact is, however, that there wasn't much fat to go around. In their seminal article entitled "Paleolithic

Nutrition" (*New England Journal of Medicine*, January 31, 1985), researchers S. Boyd Eaton, MD, and Melvin Konner, PhD, reported that, unlike today's fatted livestock, the average animal killed and eaten by our Paleolithic forebears was extremely lean. They were probably no different than animals living today in Africa, which Konner and Eaton report have only 3.9 percent body fat. The total calories derived from fat from such an animal is no more than 20 to 25 percent, which meant that there wasn't a lot of fat on the animals our forebears ate. (Compare that to today's average hamburger, which derives 50 percent of its calories from fat.)

Not only were the animals lean, but they weren't exactly easy to catch. Remember that we were not the greatest hunters in the early part of our existence. It wasn't until some 50,000 years ago that *Homo habilis*, designated by anthropologists as the "tool-maker," emerged. Before him and her, we very likely had to track and run down small game, or get larger animals to fall into deep crevices where they would be killed.

Dr. A. S. Truswell, professor emeritus of the Department of Nutrition and Food Science at the University of Sydney has studied the !Kung of Botswana, a people who have maintained their traditional ways of living and eating since Paleolithic times. Truswell points out that it takes the !Kung women four hours to gather 1,000 calories of plant foods from the forest. On the other hand, it takes men ten hours to capture the calorie equivalent in fresh game meat.

Over time, we developed a genetic predisposition to eat as much as possible, whenever possible—a behavior Robert Pritikin, in his book *The Pritikin Weight Loss Breakthrough* (Dutton Books, 1998) termed "the fat instinct." For more than a millennia, nature has equipped us with a genetic drive to eat as much food as possible, whenever it is presented to us—and to instinctively choose fat in order to maximize our calorie intake.

Of course, during ancient times, nature herself protected us from diseases of overnutrition by limiting the food supply and the amount of fat we could obtain. She gave us an abundance of low-calorie plant foods, and supplemented them with animal foods that were low in fat. That, in all probability, was the diet we evolved on, and the one we are still best suited to consume.

The problem we face today is that nature no longer controls the food supply. At least in the West, and at this moment in history, farming has triumphed over the vicissitudes of nature. The result is an abundance of food, a great percentage of which is loaded with fat and, thanks to food processing, packed with calories.

The great accomplishments of modern humans—our ability to create an abundant food supply and our increasing release from manual labor—is, to a great degree, working against our genetic design. Although we cannot go back in time, we must, in a certain sense, re-create the eating patterns of our ancestors if we are to restore our health and survive as a species. That means eating far more whole, unprocessed plant foods and limiting the quantities of animal foods, especially those rich in saturated fat. At the same time, we must increase our physical activity. To our ancestors, daily life was an enormous physical struggle simply to stay alive. For us, physical activity must be conscious forms of exercise.

As the following chapters of this book reveal, virtually all of the illnesses we face today, especially those having the most widespread and devastating effects on our health, arise from lifestyles that are in conflict with our basic genetic design. As science delves ever deeper into the human genome, and we discover more about the mysterious workings of our cells, we learn that health is founded on a clear and fairly intractable set of behaviors. When we run afoul of those behaviors, we suffer the consequences. The good news is that even after we become ill, those same behaviors, like a powerful form of medicine, can restore us to health.

· 5 ·

Mending the Heart

As toxic and as dangerous as insulin resistance is, it rarely if ever appears alone. Much more common is for it to appear with its standard accomplice, inflammation.

In truth, inflammation usually arises first. As the condition worsens, it forms the foundation for its Siamese twin, insulin resistance. Together they form the basis for an array of serious illnesses, including heart disease, cancer, diabetes, and Alzheimer's.

In the strictest sense, inflammation is nothing more than the immune system's assault on a threat to your health. Coined by the ancient Greeks to mean "a fire within," the term inflammation describes the outward symptoms of that assault—heat, fever, redness, and swelling. Some or all of these symptoms emerge when your immune system is busy attacking a disease-causing agent, such as a bacteria or virus. That attack is an altogether good thing. In fact, it's one of the reasons we have survived as a species. But like any attack, we don't want it to go on for too long.

Under healthy conditions, the immune system's reaction to any given threat is ferocious, effective, and relatively short lived. The immune system is designed to identify a problem, destroy it, and then stand down, thus resuming a state of cool quiescence. Unfortunately, that doesn't happen for most of us.

The problem today is that our blood, organs, lymph system, and joints are so filled with toxic substances that our immune systems are constantly attacking a multitude of dastardly invaders. If our immune systems could talk, they would tell us that there are just too many battles to fight. As with any war zone, there's significant collateral damage. The system is attacking the bad guys, but during those attacks, it can deform or destroy otherwise healthy tissue.

One such example occurs when your immune system attacks the LDL cholesterol particles that infiltrate the tissues of your arteries. Immune cells attempt to destroy the LDL particles, but in the process cause the artery tissue to become swollen and filled with atherosclerotic plaques that can lead to a heart attack and stroke.

Inflammation occurs in tissues throughout the body. When it occurs in the brain, it can lead to dementia and Alzheimer's disease. Elsewhere, it can lead to colon, breast, and prostate cancers, as well as diabetes, rheumatoid arthritis, diabetes, asthma, glaucoma, kidney disease, blindness, and many other serious disorders.

The realization that the immune system plays a pivotal role in the onset of most degenerative diseases has given scientists new insights into today's major killers. For years, scientists knew that people with rheumatoid arthritis and even gingivitis had higher rates of heart disease, even when their cholesterol levels were normal. They also knew that people with diabetes had higher rates of Alzheimer's. What possibly could be the connection between gingivitis and heart disease?, physicians asked—or for that matter, diabetes and Alzheimer's? That link is their common root: inflammation, which can deform joints and swell gums, and at the same time, destroy arteries and brain tissue.

The most widespread of those conditions, of course, is cardiovascular disease (illnesses of the heart and arteries), which afflicts approximately seventy million Americans, and kills about a million of us each year. Heart disease has been the number one killer since 1900 (the sole exception was 1918, when influenza and pneumonia topped the killer charts). Heart disease kills an American every thirty-four seconds, and 2,500 of us each day.

Grim as these statistics may be, they're going to get worse. More than one million American teenagers have metabolic syndrome, a primary risk factor for heart disease. If that trend continues—and most experts believe it will—the illness will afflict about ninety million Americans by the year 2010.

METABOLIC SYNDROME IS DEFINED BY THE FOLLOWING CHARACTERISTICS:

1. Abdominal obesity or increased waist circumference
2. Elevated triglycerides and low HDL cholesterol
3. Elevated blood pressure
4. Elevated inflammatory markers, such as C-reactive protein and LDL cholesterol

---

The word emergency doesn't come close to describing what we will face, both in terms of the sheer suffering and the out-of-control health care costs that the illness is causing.

This is where we must begin our investigation to learn how inflammation and insulin resistance combine to create the most deadly illnesses affecting us today, and how they can be prevented and overcome.

SLOW AND TASTY SUICIDE

At Columbia University College of Physicians and Surgeons in New York City, Mehmet Oz, MD, famed professor of surgery, author, and frequent medical guru to Oprah Winfrey and her guests, has seen pretty much everything there is to see on the inside of the human body. He is particularly knowledgeable of the workings of the heart and arteries, serving as director of the Cardiovascular Institute at Columbia University Medical Center. Dr. Oz puts the story of heart disease succinctly. "To understand heart disease, you've got to understand inflammation first, and insulin resistance second," he says. "Inflammation is really the destruction of the body by friendly fire. Our own immune system is turned against us, which is pretty scary when you realize just how powerful that system is."

The irony is that we are the ones turning that system against ourselves. We do it with behaviors that so many of us take for granted, like eating a few hamburgers each week, piling on some french fries, and topping them off with some rich desserts.

Hamburgers and french fries—not to mention many desserts—

are loaded with saturated fat, which raises the bad cholesterol in your blood, the type known as LDL (low-density lipoprotein). Once these foods and others like them are consumed, particles of LDL come flying into your blood stream and migrate onto your artery walls. In small amounts, those LDL particles would pass safely in and out of the arteries. But when LDL becomes elevated in your blood, those particles enter your arteries and get stuck inside the walls, like too many fat men trying to get out of a single doorway at the same time. The LDL piles up inside the artery tissue and then undergoes a most unfortunate change—it becomes oxidized.

Simply put, oxidation is decay. The molecules inside the LDL break up, lose electrons, and become unstable, forming new chemical arrangements that kill or deform cells, tissues, and organs. Oxidation is the process that makes skin wrinkle, organs shrink, milk sour, apples brown, and iron rust. It is what most of us call aging.

In the body, oxidation can turn healthy cells and tissues into nonfunctioning scar tissue, or cholesterol plaques, or even cancer cells and tumors. It's something like the *Invasion of the Body Snatchers,* in which healthy cells are turned into destructive ones. Your immune system recognizes the problem and realizes that it's got to do something about it.

"The body is binary," says Dr. Oz. "It's either quiescent or inflamed. If the immune system senses that something bad is happening, it sends out the storm troopers, which are macrophage cells, to take it out." And that's where inflammation starts.

Macrophages are very powerful immune cells that are sent into the artery walls, where they start gobbling up the decaying LDL particles. Unfortunately, once they've got the LDL inside their stomachs, the macrophages become bloated and poisoned, and eventually die.

Once the macrophages are neutralized, they too accumulate inside the walls of the artery. Before they die, they send out an SOS message to the rest of the immune system. They do this by producing cytokines, chemical messengers that contact the immune system's generals, which are called CD4 cells. "Send in reinforcements," the macrophages signal. "There's too much LDL here." Thanks to the cytokines, more macrophages arrive, eat the LDL, get sick, and accumulate inside the artery wall, causing the artery to become swollen and hard. This robs the artery of its normal flexibility, preventing it from expanding when the body needs to send more blood to the heart and other organs.

Complicating the problem is the fact that macrophages release oxidants as a way to kill disease-causing invaders, such as bacteria or viruses. In this setting, however, the release of oxidants only backfires: They promote the decay of LDL particles in the artery, which means that more immune cells must be called to the battle zone. There, the macrophages engorge more LDL and are poisoned and destroyed.

"Inflammation is the rusting of your arteries," says Dr. Oz succinctly. For tissue that needs to be flexible and capable of rapid expansion, arteries cannot afford to rust.

Let's say that you climb a flight of stairs, or suddenly experience stress. The heart immediately starts pumping more blood to the system. Under normal circumstances, the arteries would suddenly dilate to allow more blood to flow to the cells and the heart itself. Unfortunately, the hardened arteries cannot expand as extensively as they formerly could. With increased blood flow comes more pressure within the arterial system. It's not unlike squeezing a garden hose while the water is running.

As pressure within the artery increases, tiny cracks and fissures break open inside the inner linings of the arteries. This same cracking and fissuring can occur elsewhere such as the kidneys or eyes, thus damaging these organs as well. When the pressure becomes great enough, arteries can burst open. If that happens in the brain, a stroke occurs. If it takes place in the heart, a heart attack can ensue.

But even if an artery doesn't rupture, it still has open wounds that are exposed to infiltration by decaying LDL particles and attacking immune cells, both of which combine to create more inflammation in the artery wall.

We continue eating those hamburgers, fried chicken, fatty desserts, or nachos and cheese, all of which are rich in saturated fat. That means that the LDL particles keep coming, and the macrophages keep eating the poison.

Once they've become engorged with LDL, the macrophages are called *foam cells*—they are literally foamy with LDL bloating. Eventually, they become so numerous that they break through the tile-like inner lining of the artery wall, called the *endothelial layer*, which is where the blood flows, forming a fatty streak.

"The problem is made worse when homocysteine shows up and acts like acid on that endothelial layer," Dr. Oz points out. Homocysteine is a highly corrosive amino acid that reaches dangerous levels when we eat too much red meat, dairy products, eggs, and chicken—in short, animal proteins. These proteins elevate levels of the amino acid methionine, which is converted into homocysteine, an amino acid that acts like acid rain on the delicate endothelial tissue.

"The inside lining of the artery is like Teflon," says Dr. Oz. "It creates a smooth surface so that blood can easily pass through the artery. Homocysteine burns away some of that surface to expose the medial layer below the Teflon coating. Once it's exposed, it attracts more LDL particles and immune cells. That medial layer is electrically charged. So the result is something like a thunderstorm inside your arteries."

Your body responds to a wound inside your artery wall in much the same way as it does to a wound anywhere else in the body. The liver is ordered via chemical messengers to produce clotting proteins that combine with blood platelets to form a Band-Aid over the open wound. In order for that Band-Aid to be created, clotting proteins chemically join to form a sticky substance called *fibrinogen*, which is a kind of glue that binds platelets together. The sticky platelets form a scab over the wound and thus begin the healing process.

Unfortunately for too many of us today, the liver overproduces clotting proteins, which in turn make too much fibrinogen. These cause the blood to become sticky, which in turn causes platelets to clump together and form clots within the blood. Those blood clots can be big enough to reduce the flow of blood to the heart, brain, or other organs. They can also break free from the wound in the artery, float downstream, and get lodged in a smaller vessel, where they can block blood flow entirely to a vital organ.

There are numerous reasons why the liver overproduces fibrinogen, and most of them are related to lifestyle choices. One of the big ones, of course, is cigarette smoking, which causes drastic changes in the liver. The liver responds by producing higher levels of fibrinogen, which increases the likelihood of blood clots. Other reasons include a lack of exercise, too much homocysteine in the blood, and chronic infections, including such seemingly benign conditions as gingivitis. Still another is the consumption of a high-fat diet. Recently, scientists found that hormone replacement therapy (HRT) also elevates fibrinogen. This may well be the reason why HRT is associated with greater risk of heart attack in some women.

Contrary to what many believe, heart disease is the number one killer of women (many assume it's breast cancer). More than nine million women suffer from coronary heart disease and each year 50,000 women die of the illness (as compared to 40,500 who die from breast cancer).

All of us can reduce fibrinogen levels—and inflammation overall—with daily exercise, cessation of smoking (if you do smoke), and a reduction in consumption of animal protein and saturated fats. (The program described in chapter 12 can dramatically reduce inflammation overall and fibrinogen specifically.)

One of the problems with poor lifestyle choices is that they are consistent—we tend to eat the same foods each day and engage in the same level of activity, or the lack of it. Consequently, LDL continues to pour into the blood, which means foam cells continue to accumulate inside the artery. Eventually, they form a fatty streak inside the artery, which, if the conditions go unchanged, will grow into a full blown plaque, a condition known as *atherosclerosis*. Inside the plaque, tiny puddles of cholesterol lie in the bellies of the macrophages. Eventually, the stomachs of the macrophages burst open and release that cholesterol. Over time, the tiny puddles form larger pools of cholesterol inside the plaque. As they do, they make the plaque unstable and force it to eventually erupt, much like a boil. It spews forth its inner contents into the blood stream and leaves behind a wound in the artery wall.

The body responds to this latest wound by sending more fibrinogen and blood platelets. But now the conditions are ripe for a much more dangerous event. The plaque is larger; there's more fibrinogen; the blood platelets are stickier, and prone to form an even larger clot. A large clot not only can block the artery entirely; more likely, it can break free, float downstream, and block blood flow to the heart or brain, thus causing a heart attack or stroke.

Interestingly, the National Heart, Lung, and Blood Institute—the cardiovascular wing of the National Institutes of Health—has reported that most heart attacks occur in people with relatively small plaques that block only 30 percent or less of the artery. That means it isn't the size of the plaque that's so dangerous, but the plaque's tendency to rupture, along with the blood's tendency to form large clots. It's the clots that block blood flow to the heart and bring on a heart attack.

As if all of this were not bad enough, insulin resistance actually makes it worse.

GASOLINE ON THE FIRE

Eric Topol, MD, now at Scripps Health Clinic in San Diego County, California, is one of the giants of modern medicine. He was chairman of the Department of Cardiovascular Medicine and Genetics at Case Western Reserve University, and the Chief Academic

Officer and Chairman of the Department of Cardiovascular Medicine at the Cleveland Clinic. He has more than 950 original scientific publications under his name and he's edited eighteen books, including the *Textbook of Interventional Cardiology*. Even if you've never been treated at the Cleveland Clinic, you have probably heard Topol's name in the news. He's the man largely responsible for blowing the whistle on Merck & Co. for the hidden dangers associated with its pain medication Vioxx. Topol accused Merck of scientific misconduct, misrepresenting facts, and endangering patients. Eventually, Merck had to pull the drug from the market and was forced to pay enormous fines for misleading consumers.

Contrary to what you might think about a person of such preeminent status, Topol is soft spoken, friendly, and open. Physically lean and precise with his words, he nonetheless seems utterly relaxed in conversation and even enjoys going over the basic science that explains how we find ourselves in the current health crisis.

"There isn't any question that insulin resistance is epidemic and contributes to heart disease," he begins, "in part because obesity rates are climbing. Overweight and obesity take people over the edge and cause a breakdown in many different areas of the body, including the function and health of the heart and arteries."

Insulin resistance and inflammation are joined in our fat tissue, says Dr. Topol. The more your insulin levels rise, and stay high, the more overweight you become. Adipose tissue is a highly active organ producing an array of inflammatory cytokines, including tumor necrosis factor (TNF) and interleukin-6 (IL-6). When secreted in higher than normal quantities, these chemicals degrade cells and tissues, most likely by oxidizing fat cells. Tumor necrosis factor alone degrades the membranes of cells throughout the body and increases the risk of insulin resistance. Studies have shown that TNF plays a central role in the onset of diabetes. Virtually everyone who is overweight has higher levels of TNF in their bloodstreams.

Whenever a person is in insulin resistance, he's unable to burn all the glucose in his bloodstream. Forced to get rid of the excess blood sugar, the body converts it to fat and stores it as adipose tissue. That means that if you're insulin resistant, you're making more fat, and if you're making more fat, you're making more TNF and IL-6.

When cells are attacked by these inflammatory cytokines, the body calls out the macrophages to help eliminate the deformed cells and the high levels of TNF and IL-6. Once macrophages show up on the scene, however, they release more oxidants, which cause even greater damage and higher levels of inflammation.

TNF and IL-6 do not simply stay in the adipose tissue, however. They flow into the bloodstream and make their way to the main arteries, including the coronary arteries that lead to the heart. There they degrade artery tissue and add to the inflammation that's already taking place.

At that point, another group of cells arrives on the scene—these called *adhesion molecules*. For a long time, scientists believed that these molecules were essentially the glue that held together ligaments, muscles, and just about everything else in the body. That alone is a pretty important job, but recent research has revealed that these tiny chemicals are involved in a lot of other activities as well, including directing the immune system's efforts to heal wounds, including the wounds that occur in the arteries.

"Adhesion molecules are already present because the artery has been wounded by several factors, including by homocysteine and high blood pressure," says Dr. Topol. "They're already trying to repair the endothelium."

Adhesion molecules are the body's Velcro. They're sticky. Once inside the artery, they start gluing all the chemical players together—TNF, IL-6, LDL, homocysteine, macrophages, platelets, you name it. That means that all of these highly inflammable substances are stuck inside the artery tissue, like a big crowd in an elevator. Something's got to give—and that something is often the artery wall itself. An even bigger, bulging plaque emerges, one that protrudes into the inner pathway of the artery. Moreover, these conditions, which only escalate, make the plaque more volatile and prone to rupture. The more rupturing of plaque, the more at risk you are of creating a large clot that can trigger a heart attack or stroke.

ADIPONECTIN: ONE OF THE BODY'S MOST IMPORTANT HEALERS

At this point, things may look pretty grim, but the body is nonetheless capable of producing substances that can come to the rescue. One of the most important of these is *adiponectin*.

Adiponectin is an anti-inflammatory hormone that can restore insulin sensitivity, and get all of those crowded cells, LDL, and cytokines out of the elevator. Once it arrives on the scene of the wound, adiponectin immediately sends out cytokines that communicate with all the many chemical and cellular players that are combining to cause the damage. Acting as a kind of traffic cop, the adiponectin orders the body to produce fewer adhesion molecules, thus allowing more of the inflammatory chemicals to pass freely from the site. It cools the effects of the macrophages by suppressing their tendency to consume the TNF and other inflammatory chemicals in the area. Adiponectin also induces apoptosis in some cells that may cause additional problems in the healing of the artery wall. And finally, it increases insulin sensitivity. In fact, it is so good at this job that some studies have shown that high levels of adiponectin alone are enough to take people out of insulin resistance.

There's a catch, however. The body can only produce adiponectin from lean adipocytes—small fat cells. In other words, you've got to be at a normal or healthy weight to produce sufficient quantities of adiponectin in order to take you out of insulin resistance. People who are overweight or obese produce lower amounts of adiponectin, and more TNF and IL-6, which is one possible explanation why people with insulin resistance and hyperinsulinemia (elevated insulin) do not heal as quickly as those who are not insulin resistant.

The good news is that as people lose weight, their adiponectin production increases, which in turn provides all the positive effects of this powerful hormone. Scientists are searching for ways to create new drugs that will increase adiponectin levels in insulin-resistant people, and thus decrease their risk of heart disease. (As we will see in the next chapter, adiponectin is a powerful protector against cancer, as well.)

Yet another safeguard in the body's fight against heart disease is HDL cholesterol, or high-density lipoprotein, otherwise known as the good cholesterol. HDL has exactly the opposite effect on arteries as LDL. Rather than bring cholesterol into the artery wall, HDL shepherds it away from the artery and over to the liver, where it is converted to a water-soluble substance and eliminated from the body through the feces.

HDL also acts as an antioxidant, preventing the decay of LDL and thus slowing the atherosclerotic process.

Fiber also assists in the process by binding with fats, including saturated fats, in the gut and then eliminating them from the body. The more fiber in the diet, the less saturated fat goes into the liver. That means less LDL goes into the bloodstream.

The National Heart, Lung, and Blood Institute (NHLBI) urges people to adopt a diet and lifestyle that will keep LDL levels below 100 mg/dl (milligrams per deciliter of blood). But Dr. Topol says that that number should go even lower.

"There are societies in Asia and Africa that have LDL levels below 70 mg/dl," says Dr. Topol. "And they don't suffer heart attacks. So I think that LDL number of 100 is a little high to feel safe. I'd like to see it at 70 or lower. In fact, we really haven't seen the LDL number be too low at this point."

As for HDL, the NHLBI recommends 60 mg/dl or higher. In the past, the U.S. Surgeon General recommended an HDL level of 40, but recent government agencies have urged people to go even higher.

It's essential that we do all we can to raise our HDL levels. Here are eleven ways to do that—and reduce inflammation overall—without any drug intervention.

1. Eat antioxidant-rich whole grains, vegetables, and fruits. A British study reported that drinking three cups of orange juice a day increased HDL levels by 21 percent during a

period of three weeks. Orange juice, of course, is just one of many plant sources of antioxidants. Not only will antioxidant-rich foods boost your HDL, but they will bind with saturated fats and lower your LDL.

2. Eat niacin-rich foods, which include salmon, trout, nuts, beans, leafy greens, the white meat of chicken, the white meat of turkey, and peanut butter. Ask your doctor to monitor any use of niacin supplements, especially because they can be harmful to some people at even moderate doses.

3. Avoid sugar and other processed foods, which increase weight and insulin resistance, and lower HDL.

4. Eat soy foods, such as soybeans, tofu, tempeh, miso, tamari, and shoyu. Soy foods reduce LDL and triglycerides, while boosting HDL.

5. Exercise daily. A thirty-minute walk, or some other form of aerobic exercise, can significantly boost your HDL.

6. Lose weight. As we've already seen, excess weight increases triglycerides and LDL, while lowering HDL. Conversely, weight loss boosts HDL levels.

7. Drink alcohol in moderation. Studies have shown that moderate amounts of alcohol (one or two drinks per day) can increase HDL, especially if it is drunk during a meal. Some research suggests that alcohol consumed during a meal may move cholesterol deposits out of the artery wall.

8. If you smoke, stop.

9. Eat onions, which some researchers now believe can significantly elevate HDL.

10. Eat cooked grains that contain soluble fiber, such as oatmeal, brown rice, and apples, grapes, and citrus fruits. These

foods lower LDL and after regular consumption for approximately three months raise HDL as well.

11. Eat healthful oils from such sources as nuts (almonds, Brazil, and walnuts), and olive and sesame oils. As we saw in the previous chapter, polyunsaturated and monounsaturated fats speed the burning of adipose fat, enhance weight loss, create satiety, and boost immune function. They can also lower LDL and raise HDL levels.

Another test that Dr. Topol and other authorities recommend we have is called C-reactive protein (CRP), which measures overall inflammation that may be occurring throughout the body. C-reactive protein is produced in the liver. When the liver is inflamed, due to the production of inflammatory compounds produced in the liver or elsewhere in the body, C-reactive protein levels rise. Like LDL and HDL, C-reactive protein can be measured with a simple blood test. Safe levels are 0.5 mg/dl or lower.

Other important tests and risk factors that you should know are as follows:

- Triglycerides, or blood fats, should be no higher than 150 mg/dl, and preferably much lower.
- Homocysteine: Normal ranges from 4 to 12 micromoles per liter of blood (expressed as μmol/l), but cardiologists routinely request that it be 10 μmol/L or lower.
- Fibrinogen: Normal ranges from 200 to 400 mg/dl, but most cardiologists like to see it well below 350 mg/dl.
- Total cholesterol should be below 150 mg/dl, but as Dr. Topol points out, cardiologists now view total cholesterol as largely

insignificant, since the LDL is the primary cholesterol culprit, and total cholesterol does not reveal exactly what the LDL number really is.

The program described in chapter 12 will help you get all of your numbers well into these ranges.

• • •

Heart disease is the greatest killer today, but ironically it is the most preventable illness we face. By addressing the underlying causes of the illness—inflammation and insulin resistance—we can not only wipe out heart disease, but we can also reduce our risk of diabetes, cancer, Alzheimer's, and so many other threats to our lives.

· 6 ·

Preventing and Reversing
the Spread of Cancer

The path that leads to cancer is an insidious one. Believe it or not, it even has its pleasures. For many of us, the first sign that we're on that path is a symptom that we take for granted today—weight gain. You put on a few pounds, and then a few more, and before you know it you're twenty or thirty pounds overweight. The rise in weight is often the butt of jokes, and is considered by many to be a normal consequence of aging. But the changes taking place in the liver, blood, and in your cells are anything but normal. Even more dangerous, these changes, in most cases, do not cause overt symptoms. On the contrary, they occur secretly, silently, until the day when the malignant cells are able to override the immune and health-supporting systems, which is when you finally know you are in trouble.

What we don't realize is that many of the changes that lead to cancer—especially the most common cancers, such as breast, prostate, colon, lung, endometrial, and ovarian cancers—are driven by insulin. It's true, other factors play important roles in the onset of many cancers, but insulin is still among the driving forces in the vast majority of them, even in cases where hormones and *oncogenes* (genes that transform healthy cells into cancer) are clearly implicated. Insulin is a known *mitogen*, meaning it triggers the reproduction of cells and the growth of tissues. Cancer needs insulin to thrive. And in an insulin-resistant environment, it gets plenty of what it needs.

Your insulin levels are controlled largely by the foods you eat every day and the amount of exercise you do. For decades, scientists have pointed to certain foods as promoters of cancer, or as actual causes of the illness. Clear associations between foods rich in fat, or highly processed foods, and certain types of cancer were established long ago. In the same way, researchers have shown again and again that exercise is associated with a lower risk of cancer. The problem has been that many of the biological links between cancer and lifestyle factors remained unknown. Today, much of that is changing, as is our understanding of how this disease comes about.

Increasingly, scientists are seeing the onset of cancer as a series of stages in a degenerative process. At the early stages, lack of exercise and certain foods, especially those rich in calories and fat, combine to create a set of very harmful disorders—specifically, insulin resistance, weight gain, metabolic syndrome, and chronic, low-grade inflammation. From there, things get worse. These disorders themselves release a horde of poisonous substances that change the way cells behave and function. Eventually, they can alter gene function and form the basis for a malignancy.

This is why our understanding of insulin, insulin resistance, metabolic syndrome, and inflammation is so important: because these factors are often the underlying conditions that alter cellular and genetic behavior and form the basis for cancer. Many of our daily behaviors create these conditions. However, once these disorders are in place, they set off a series of events—a kind of domino effect—that gradually poisons the body, destroys our defenses, and leads to malignancy.

Just as we help create these disorders, we also have the power to reverse them. We can cool inflammation and overcome metabolic syndrome—and in the process, restore our health. For those who are already diagnosed with cancer, changing these underlying conditions can dramatically extend life and improve chances of survival.

CAUSES OF CANCER

We have all been conditioned to see cigarette smoking as bad for our health, but we think nothing of giving children a big bag of candy—the "goody bag"—or feeding them a diet consisting of hamburgers, french fries, and soda. These foods have an addictive effect on all of us, no matter what our age. Indeed, they are even seen by most of us as "the normal way to eat." Yet the human body does not consider these foods to be normal, or healthy. The high-fat, highly processed diet is only some sixty years old, and unlike anything we have eaten in human experience. Moreover, a lifestyle without physical activity—even moderate exertion—is unlike anything our ancestors knew. But more important, the daily behaviors that we take for granted inevitably lead to inflammation, insulin resistance, and—if allowed to go far enough— metabolic syndrome.

Tens of millions of Americans have allowed the degeneration to go on for too long. One in four adult Americans—forty million Americans—have metabolic syndrome, which is characterized by overweight (especially around the middle), high insulin, high blood glucose, high LDL cholesterol, high triglycerides, high blood pressure, inflammation, and low HDL cholesterol. In people over sixty, the percentage is 40 percent—nearly half! Metabolic syndrome is a prediabetic state, which means that it increases the risk of all the disorders associated with diabetes, such as blindness, kidney disease, poor circulation, gout, infections, and gangrenous limbs. But the effects of metabolic syndrome go far beyond these disorders. Those with metabolic syndrome have much higher rates of heart disease, Alzheimer's, and many common cancers including those of the breast, prostate, colon, and lung. U.K. researchers reviewed data from more than 140 studies and found that overweight is linked to increased risk of both common and less common types of cancer. More than 280,000 cases were reviewed of more than 20 different types of cancer. There were strong correlations between an overweight and in throat, thyroid, colon, kidney, endometrial, and other cancers.

It's easy to see why this disorder is so threatening to health: The body is flooded with poisons—high cholesterol, insulin, glucose, triglycerides—as well as suffering from high blood pressure. These toxins and disorders, in turn, lead to high levels of inflammation, which releases an overabundance of free radicals in the blood and tissues. Free radicals, or oxidants, are highly reactive oxygen molecules that, in most cases, simply kill cells, but in many instances deform them. Very often, those deformed cells combine to form scar tissue, or nonfunctioning tissue that can appear anywhere in the body. Cataracts are but one example of the scarring caused by oxidants in the bloodstream. In a high-oxidant environment, hordes of free radicals bombard DNA, killing many cells and causing mutations in others. Some of those mutations can trigger the onset of cancer.

And then there is the added burden of too much body weight, which is created in part by high insulin levels. When blood sugar becomes too high, the body converts those sugars into blood fats, triglycerides. Insulin then forces those triglycerides into fat cells, thus making us fatter.

Adipose tissue—ordinary body fat—is highly active, producing an array of cytokines. When we are overweight, that fatty tissue produces many destructive cytokines, including tumor necrosis factor and IL-6.

"Fat cells are very active," said Pinchas Cohen, MD, pediatric endocrinologist at the University of California Los Angeles (UCLA) Medical Center in Santa Monica. "There's lots of products going out of them, and most of them are bad." One of the more dangerous by-products of fat cells is the female hormone estrogen, which at high levels can be extremely toxic.

Estrogen is an important factor in both the cause and maintenance of breast and prostate cancers. At high levels, estrogen can act like growth hormone, causing tissue to grow rapidly in hormone-sensitive organs such as the breast, uterus, ovaries, and prostate. These growing tissues can block blood and lymph vessels in these organs, causing blood and waste products to accumulate and stagnate. At the same time, rising estrogen levels can also be highly inflammatory. (During ovulation, when estrogen is surging, women often suffer from swollen, inflamed, and painful breasts.) Sometimes, these inflammatory conditions alter DNA and trigger the onset of cancer.

These are some of the reasons why overweight and obese people have many times the risk of cancer of those who maintain normal, healthy weights.

A study published in the April 24, 2003, *New England Journal of Medicine* reported that overweight dramatically increases the risk of most common cancers, including those of the breast, prostate, uterus, ovaries, cervix, colon, rectum, kidneys, esophagus, liver, gall bladder, pancreas, stomach, and those of the lymph system (non-Hodgkin's lymphoma). Another study, published in the December 10, 1990, vol. 82, *Journal of the National Cancer Institute,* reported that overweight and obese women have twice the risk of contracting breast cancer than women who are at their ideal weight or lower. Unfortunately, overweight triggers cancer in other ways as well.

Expanding fat cells produce a lot of "bad" products, as Dr. Cohen so aptly put it. On the other hand, lean adipose tissue does something extremely important—it creates adiponectin, a substance that actually fights cancer. Adiponectin is one of the heroes inside our bodies. Among the many things it does is prevent blood vessels from connecting to tumors. Thus, it deprives tumors of the blood and oxygen that are essential for their survival. This talent, referred to by scientists as *antiangiogenesis,* is considered one of the Rosetta Stones in cancer research. Scientists are searching feverishly for ways to trigger antiangiogenesis—which, in essence, would give them the ability to isolate tumors and cut off their blood supply, thus causing them to die.

Remarkably, adiponectin also triggers apoptosis in cancer cells. Animal studies, including one published in the *Proceedings of the*

National Academy of Sciences (February 24, 2004), reported that not only did "adiponectin remarkably prevent new blood vessel growth" to tumors, but it also triggered a "cascade activation" that led to cancer cell death, and "significantly inhibits primary tumor growth." Finally, adiponectin significantly increases insulin sensitivity in cells, which means it helps take the body out of insulin resistance.

Clearly, higher levels of adiponectin in the bloodstream are desirable. And the way to get it is, very simply, weight loss. As weight goes up, adiponectin levels go down, thus increasing our vulnerability to all the diseases and disorders it protects us from. On the other hand, when weight drops, adiponectin levels rise, thus providing protection from cancers and other diseases caused by cells multiplying unchecked.

The protection provided by adiponection may be one of the reasons why studies have shown that women with breast cancer who lose weight live longer and have lower rates of recurrence. One such study, done by Dr. James Hebert and his colleagues at the University of Massachusetts (UMass) Medical School showed that women with breast cancer who are overweight, or who gain weight after diagnosis, experience much shorter survival than those who eat a low-glycemic diet and lose weight. The study, reported in *Breast Cancer Research and Treatment* (September 1999), showed that for every 1,000 additional calories consumed, there was an 84 percent increased risk of recurrence. Those women who ate the most calories and had the highest rates of recurrence got most of those additional calories from fat. Hebert and his coworkers found that just eating an additional 100 calories per day over the standard 1,200 calorie diet increased the risk of recurrence by 5 percent.

Low adiponectin levels may be especially dangerous to women

for another reason: They are associated with a particularly powerful form of cancer. A study done by Japanese researchers and published in *Clinical Cancer Research* in November 2003, reported the following:

> Results suggest that the low serum (blood) adiponectin levels are significantly associated with an increased risk of breast cancer and that tumors arising in women with the low serum adiponectin levels are more likely to show biologically aggressive phenotype. The association between obesity and breast cancer risk might be partly explained by adiponectin.

Adiponectin has been found to play a role in a wide array of cancers, including those of the colon, rectum, prostate, and endometrium.

The good news is that adiponectin levels can be restored rapidly, usually within weeks of adopting a diet and lifestyle that causes weight loss.

INSULIN AND GROWTH HORMONES—
A TOXIC COCKTAIL

The human body is an awesome symphony of chemical and cellular functions, each one dependent on many others to remain in balance and in health. At the center of that symphony is insulin.

Insulin is itself a mitogen, a substance that stimulates cells to replicate. Scientists have shown that when elevated, insulin can act as a trigger and actually fuel cancer proliferation. A good example is the BCL2 gene, now recognized as one of the genetic causes of several types of cancers, including breast cancer. Not all women who have the Bcl-2 gene get cancer. But those who have the gene and maintain high insulin levels are at much greater risk. Why?

When high blood levels of insulin are sustained over time, cells can develop a specialized BCL2 receptor on the cell membrane. And in an insulin-resistant environment, BCL2 receptors proliferate. That receptor, which acts as an antenna for the swarming insulin in the blood, is linked directly to the BCL2 gene inside the cell's DNA. Once insulin catalyzes or phosphorylates the receptor, it lights up a kinase cascade that turns on the BCL2 gene, which in turn initiates the cancer.

Women who maintain normal or healthy insulin levels are less likely to have the BCL2 receptor. This may explain one of the reasons why women who are overweight have much higher rates of breast cancer than those who are lean. High insulin levels create weight gain; they also stimulate the BCL2 receptor.

When elevated, insulin causes the liver to produce more growth hormone, including a specific type known as *insulin-like growth factor* (IGF-1). In youth, growth hormones including IGF-1 become elevated in order to promote physical development and create normal-size adults. But as we age, we don't need as much growth hormone any more and, consequently, the body reduces its production of IGF-1 and other growth factors. This is important because growth hormone causes cells to multiply and tissue to get larger—which is exactly what a nascent cancer needs in order to become a full-blown malignancy. Growth factors trigger cell division and multiplication; in essence, they promote cancer. One of the ways the body keeps growth hormone low is by keeping insulin levels in check.

Keeping insulin in check was something our ancestors didn't

need to think about. Nature protected our forebears by limiting their menu and demanding lots of physical activity. No matter where humans lived, they all ate diets that were relatively low in fat, rich in unprocessed plant foods, and low in calories, which meant that it kept insulin levels low. At the same time, our ancestors were forced to maintain active lives—especially because early humans lived as hunter-gatherers and later as farmers. Physical activity burns calories and keeps insulin levels low. As insulin levels fell in adulthood, so too did growth hormone and overall weight. Few, if any, of our ancestors had to think about dieting and aerobic exercise. But modern life has created exactly the opposite conditions. Calories are high and physical activity is low. This causes insulin levels to rise, which in turn stimulates the liver to produce higher levels of growth hormones, especially IGF-1.

An ever-increasing body of evidence is showing that as insulin and IGF-1 go up, so too do the rates of breast, prostate, and colon cancers. "IGF-1 is one of the keys to cancer, especially cancers of the breast, prostate, and colon," says Dr. Cohen. "IGF-1 is a stimulator for cancer. There [are] associated data that show that as insulin levels go up, as IGF-1 goes up, so too does inflammation. These conditions also promote the generation of proinflammatory cytokines, which in turn promote numerous diseases, including cancer."

CHANGING THE INTERNAL ENVIRONMENT—AND MAKING CELLS BEHAVE DIFFERENTLY

If allowed to proliferate, cancer cells are virtually immortal, or, at the very least, will live as long as the host patient survives. Scientists are searching for ways to "reboot" p53. A UCLA researcher may have stumbled upon one of the ways to do just that.

James Barnard, PhD, a professor of physiological science at UCLA, has been studying the relationship between diet and health for more than thirty years. At sixty-nine years of age, Dr. Barnard is still strikingly fit. Tall and athletically built, Barnard was for much of his adult life a long-distance runner, but in recent years he has slowed down to a daily hour-long walk in the Southern California hills.

Among the populations of people Dr. Barnard has studied are those who come to the Pritikin Longevity Center, a center for the treatment of heart and vascular illnesses in Santa Monica, California, and Aventura, Florida. More than 100,000 people have been cared for at the medically supervised Longevity Centers, mostly for heart disease, diabetes, high blood pressure, claudication, and gout. The Centers' primary form of treatment is the use of a diet that is composed of low-fat animal foods, whole, unprocessed grains, vegetables, beans, and fruit. In addition, the daily exercise program is made up largely of walking, yoga, and other gentle forms of exertion.

Dr. Barnard, who has published more than 200 peer-reviewed papers, has been examining the before-and-after effects of the Pritikin diet and exercise program on these people. Among the many studies Barnard has done on the Pritikin participants is the effects of a low-fat, low-calorie diet and exercise on insulin, IGF-1, and prostate cancer.

In a study published in *Obesity Reviews* (November 3, 2002), Barnard and his colleagues found that men with prostate cancer who adopted an essentially low-fat, high plant-based diet experienced a dramatic drop in insulin levels and IGF-1. The men also experienced an increase in two important proteins known as IGFBP-1 and BP-2 that bind with IGF-1 and take it safely out of the body.

These findings might have been anticipated, but what Barnard also found was not. Doing blood assays, Barnard found that soon after adopting the diet and exercise program, the cancer cells in the prostate went into programmed cell death (apoptosis). Essentially, the cancer started to die.

Scientists have been searching for decades for ways to trigger apoptosis in cancer. They have long known that one of the problems with getting cancer to perform apoptosis was the degradation of p53 gene, and they have been researching how could it be revived. Barnard believes he found one of the ways to do that.

"The drop in insulin levels caused the liver to produce less IGF-1," Dr. Barnard says. "At the same time, the diet and exercise program also caused BP-1 and BP-2 to rise, causing a further drop in IGF-1. These factors created the conditions for the initiating of apoptosis in the cancer cells."

Blood changes suddenly cause the cancer to behave differently because, Dr. Barnard explains, "IGF-1 degrades the p53 gene. When IGF-1 dropped, the p53 was restored. P53 stimulates cell repair. And if the cell cannot be repaired, it tells the cell to go into apoptosis."

In further studies, Barnard found that a diet low in fat and rich in unprocessed plant foods alone brought about a drop in insulin and IGF-1, and triggered apoptosis. Interestingly, exercise alone also triggered an increase in apoptosis. When combined, diet and exercise had an even more powerful therapeutic effect, causing even greater levels of apoptosis.

Many recent studies have corroborated these findings. Increasingly, scientists are finding that appropriate diet and exercise lowers insulin and IGF-1, and brings about apoptosis in cancer cells. This new understanding may be among the reasons why Asian men have much lower rates of prostate cancer than American men do. Moreover, when Asian men suffer prostate cancer, the disease does not become a full-blown malignancy, but remains asymptomatic and confined to the prostate gland. Many Asians with prostate cancer die in old age, never knowing that they had the disease.

All high-calorie, high-protein foods, including milk products, will result in higher levels of IGF-1. Recent research has shown that men who regularly consume milk or eat dairy products have higher levels of IGF-1 and higher rates of prostate cancer.

BREAST CANCER: THE FEMALE VERSION OF PROSTATE CANCER?

Many scientists today believe that breast cancer is the female version of prostate cancer. And not surprisingly, insulin and IGF-1 are at the very heart of both diseases. Women with chronically high insulin and IGF-1 have much higher rates of breast cancer than women who have lower insulin and normal IGF-1. A study reported in the *Annals of Oncology* (October 2005), compared the eating habits of more than 2,500 women with breast cancer with 2,500 control subjects who did not have breast cancer. The researchers documented how often each of the 5,000 women ate such foods as "biscuits, brioches, cakes, and ice cream," as well as "sugar, honey, jam, marmalade, and chocolate." Their findings could almost have been predicted. As they reported in their study, "We found a direct association between breast cancer risk and consumption of sweet foods with high glycemic index and load, which increase insulin and insulin growth factors."

The glycemic index is a numerical system designed to measure the rise in blood sugar from specific foods. Processed foods, such as white bread, white rolls, pastries, and candy—just to name a few—are loaded with rapidly absorbed carbohydrates. They raise blood sugar and insulin levels rapidly and consequently have high glycemic index scores. Foods with low glycemic index scores are slowly absorbed and keep glucose and insulin levels low. Most vegetables, for example, are very low on the glycemic index.

MUTATIONS MAKE IT
MORE DIFFICULT TO TREAT CANCER

A full-blown cancer takes years—and in some cases more than a decade—to develop before it can be detected by medical instruments or physical examination. That means that a very serious disease has gone unnoticed by the immune system.

"The genius of cancer is that it hides in the body while it grows, and then it becomes increasingly difficult to treat once it can be detected," said Edmundo Muniz, MD, PhD, a former cancer researcher and now president of Tigris Pharmaceuticals. Dr. Muniz is the former vice president of Eli Lilly Research Laboratories Global Oncology program, where he helped create numerous cancer drugs, seven of which have been approved by the FDA and are now used to treat cancer patients worldwide. He is widely regarded as one of the world's leading experts on cancer and its treatment.

"In the early growth stages, cancer looks to the immune system like something created by the body, and therefore part of a natural process," he says. "This means that the immune system does not attack the cancer, because it does not recognize it as a threat. But once the cancer becomes strong enough, it overwhelms the immune system and then it is very difficult to treat."

In this way, cancer bears some similarities to HIV (human immunodeficiency virus), the basis for AIDS. "HIV learned from cancer," Dr. Muniz says. He adds:

> Viruses use the genome from cells to grow. HIV looks to the immune system like other cells. Cancer is similar in this regard. Cancer cells look to the immune system like normal cells that are in revolution. From an evolutionary point of view, revolution has often been seen as a good thing. It's a kind of advancement in our ability to survive, and therefore seen by the body, including the immune system, as a forward movement. But cancer cells do not perform any life-supporting activity. They consume the life of the body.

FAILURE TO COMMIT CELL DEATH

Once the body wakes up to the presence of cancer, it starts signaling the malignant cells to initiate programmed cell death, apoptosis. Unfortunately, the abundance of free radicals in the system have brought about mutations in the cancer cells, essentially allowing them to act independently of the overall system. One of the most important of these mutations is the degradation of a key gene known as p53.

P53 watches over cellular behavior and, when needed, tells cells to enter a phase of cellular repair. If cells cannot repair themselves, p53 orders the cell to initiate programmed cell death. One of the first things cancer does is turn off p53. That means that when neighboring cells order the cancer to either repair itself or initiate programmed cell death, it can disobey.

In addition, cancer develops certain armoring characteristics that, over time, make it more resistant to chemotherapy. In effect, it learns how to adapt to the hostile conditions of the chemotherapy, making it even more difficult to treat. This is why recurrence of cancer—that is, cancer's return after it has been forced into remission by chemotherapy—is so difficult to treat. It is actually a far more virulent disease the second time around.

NEW MEDICAL APPROACHES
TO TREATING CANCER

Not surprisingly, the advances in our understanding of cancer have led to new approaches in its treatment. Indeed, chemotherapy is now being seen as roughly analogous to Sherman's slash-and-burn march to the sea, and is already being viewed less as a cure and more as a means of gaining time. One of the shortcomings of chemotherapy, doctors recognize, is that it actually weakens the body's own efforts to fight the disease.

"Chemotherapy can slow the growth of cancer by killing cancer cells," says Dr. Muniz. "But chemotherapy kills both cancer cells and immune cells. In this way, chemotherapy is like antibiotics, which kill both bacteria and healthy cells as well. But one of the reasons antibiotics work is because they are not strong enough to kill the immune system. The immune system is still intact and can assist the work of antibiotics to kill the bacteria."

With chemotherapy, both the cancer and the immune system are weakened, but the cancer is able to rebound more rapidly, in part because the chemotherapy itself creates the conditions for the cancer's rebirth.

Once administered, chemotherapy leaves in its wake enormous quantities of free radicals, which can trigger additional mutations in DNA and bring about the rebirth of the disease. Free radicals also fire the embers of any surviving nests of old cancer, thus bringing them back to life.

"In the middle ages, people were hit by a two-by-four over the head as anesthesia so that they could extract a tooth or be operated on," says Dr. Muniz. "That's basically what we're doing with chemotherapy. Chemotherapy kills everything—the cancer and also healthy cells. In essence, we're hitting people with two-by-fours. The person is half dead and half alive from the treatment itself. And unlike the case of antibiotics, we cannot count on the immune system to help us fight the disease. Thankfully [we know so much more about cancer today] and we're moving beyond that kind of treatment."

The future will bring entirely new approaches, Dr. Muniz says. "Today we know so much more about the genetic makeup of cancer, and the person who suffers from the disease, that we can tailor a specific treatment for a person's unique genetic makeup."

Dr. Muniz says that new drugs are now being designed to directly interfere with specific kinase pathways within the cancer cell, and in the process destroy the disease. One of those pathways is known as EGF, epidermal growth factor kinase. Dr. Muniz points to two drugs, Iressa and Tarceva, now being used effectively to treat cancer. "These drugs attach to the EGF pathway and stop cell division," Dr. Muniz says. "We are finding that they are working extremely well in people with lung cancer."

Another such drug now being used successfully, Gleevec, blocks the enzyme that fuels the growth of chronic myeloid leukemia (CML). Before Gleevec, the average survival rate for people with CML was four to six years. On Gleevec, only 16 percent of patients with CML have relapsed, and many physicians believe that the drug will stretch the lifespan of people with CML up to twenty years.

Gleevec is also being used to treat people with gastrointestinal cancer, which happens to be driven by the same enzyme as CML. Prior to Gleevec, there was no effective treatment for gastrointestinal cancer, with the average patient surviving only one to two years after diagnosis. More than half the patients treated with Gleevec are currently showing no signs of disease.

The targeting of specific kinases also opens up the possibility that scientists may be able to insert specific commands to cancer cells. One of the commands scientists are most eager to insert into cancer cells is the order to commit suicide.

FOOD AS THERAPY

Scientists have learned a great deal about how foods affects us on the cellular and even genetic levels. One of the most promising of those foods is green tea. At the Medical College of Georgia, cell biologist Stephen Hsu, PhD, has been studying green tea for more than a decade. He and others have found that the antioxidant in green tea, epigallocatechin-3-gallate (EGCG), triggers the flow of protein messengers that force cancer cells to differentiate. If they are unable to do so, the antioxidant instead initiates programmed cell death.

Michael Wargovich, PhD, a long-time cancer researcher at the South Carolina Cancer Center, points out: "In tumors, certain signal pathways become corrupted and stop functioning so that the cells keep growing. It's like having the light switch taped in the 'on' position. When that happens in cells, certain functions become degraded and, in time, deplete the machinery and can cause some cells to become cancerous. Green tea reregulates the cell, it reboots the system so to speak, to accept the command to stop growing."

At the very least, green tea is worth drinking for its anti-inflammatory powers. Because most diseases today involve inflammation, green tea may provide some protection against heart disease, diabetes, arthritis, and Alzheimer's disease.

Other foods affect genes in ways that also protect us from cancer. Soybeans, and soybean products, are a good example. Soybeans, scientists have found, stimulate the activity of 123 genes in the prostate that combine to suppress inflammation, tumor growth, and initiate DNA repair. Curcumin, a substance found in the spice turmeric, inhibits genes from triggering inflammation that forms the basis for breast, colon, and prostate cancer, as well as Alzheimer's disease. The people of India are the highest per capita consumers of turmeric; they also have the lowest rates of Alzheimer's disease in the world.

David Heber, MD, PhD, director of the UCLA Center for Human Nutrition and a professor of medicine and public health at the UCLA's David Geffen School of Medicine, urges people to eat more plant foods as a way to add antioxidants and to combat inflammation. "A number of colorful fruits and vegetables have natural dietary agents that are antioxidant and anti-inflammatory," he told us in an interview. "The most evidence exists for soy protein, turmeric (which contains curcumin), resveratrol (found in red wine), pomegranate ellagitannins, tea polyphenols from green tea and black tea, aged garlic extract, and lycopene from tomato products." Dr. Heber recommends that people eat a diet of "five to nine servings per day of fruits and vegetables" in order to get adequate quantities of antioxidants and other plant chemicals that reduce inflammation.

He also points to our mental state as a powerful factor in healing. Dr. Heber recalls the experience of famed financier and former junk bond maven Michael Milken, who was diagnosed with terminal prostate cancer in 1993 and is not only still alive, but thriving and healthy.

"The most powerful immune organ in the human body is the brain and central nervous system," said Dr. Heber. "I believe that an individual can influence disease processes. I have seen too many people die within a year of the death of a spouse or within a year of retirement to discount the impact of mental function on health. We are a long way from proof, but I believe that there is an individual healing process not reflected in our large cancer studies which predict mortality. With a PSA of 24 and a Gleason score of 9 [both indicating the presence of virulent cancer], Michael Milken statistically has outlived every prediction and beaten prostate cancer. Was it his diet, his medical treatment, his mental determination, or a combination of all three?"

One of the most powerful tools we have for preventing cancer, or helping to treat it after it arises, is our insulin. Keep your insulin levels low and you will prevent or reduce insulin resistance, overweight, inflammation, and metabolic syndrome—in other words, you'll control the very disorders that lead to cancer, and fuel its growth once it manifests.

· 7 ·

Stress and Insulin

Everybody's got stress—the universal disorder. The sources of stress in our lives seem endless, but most of them are related in one way or another to time, or the lack of it. We're all in a rush to get someplace, and all too often we're late. Caught in traffic, behind on some deadline, and pushing ourselves to our limits. Remember that quaint little term that we used to apply to the latest form of technology—the "time- and labor-saving device"? The idea was that you used this piece of machinery to get a job done quickly so you could return to your leisure. The problem today is that the time you save on one project is used to catch up on another, the one that you've neglected for lack of time. Every moment, it seems, is filled, spoken for, or scheduled. And every new technological advance—e-mail is just one example—seems to steal more time and make new demands. In the twenty-first century, progress all too often means more stress.

It's taking a toll. The World Health Organization predicts that by the year 2020, stress-related disorders will be the second leading cause of death in the world. The physical and mental disorders arising from stress on the job now cost U.S. industry more than $300 billion annually in low productivity and health care costs.

Stress, especially when it's chronic, is dangerous for two reasons. First, it causes profound and often destructive changes in our biochemistry. It weakens the immune system, damages the heart, alters and in some cases destroys the neurons responsible for memory, and increases the likelihood of contracting various kinds of cancers. One of the most important ways that stress affects our health is by elevating insulin levels, and keeping them elevated, eventually resulting in weight gain, insulin resistance, and all those conditions that flow from metabolic syndrome, including diabetes.

Second, it often causes us to engage in coping behaviors that are themselves dangerous to health. People under stress are more likely to smoke cigarettes, drink alcohol to excess, and eat foods high in fat and calories. For many people, the methods used to cope with stress are as destructive as the stress itself.

Stress has become a major source of illness today, in part because it drives up insulin levels so precipitously. To combat stress we need to understand its effect on insulin levels and then determine what we can do about it.

FACING THE WOOLY MAMMOTH

Stress is really another word for fear. Implicit in every stressful situation is the recognition that something valuable is threatened. And therein lies one of the keys to understanding stress. When it comes to assessing a threat, stressful situations are in the eye of the beholder.

Sonia Lupien, PhD, is one of the world's leading experts on stress. As director of the Center for Studies of Human Stress at McGill University's Douglas Hospital Research Center in Montreal, Canada, she has studied the effects of stress on people of all age groups, from the very young to the very old. Dr. Lupien is French-Canadian and speaks English with a distinct French accent.

She presents much of her information as historical analogies and human stories, rather than the dry facts of science.

"We live in very secure countries, relatively speaking," says Dr. Lupien. "We're not living in Iraq or Darfur. Yet, according to the World Health Organization, in twenty years, most of us are going to be dying from stress-related problems. How is this possible? The answer is that the human body cannot tell the difference between an absolute stressor and a relative stressor."

An absolute stressor, according to Dr. Lupien, is a situation in which our lives are clearly in danger. Relative stressors, on the other hand, are those that threaten our status, identities, or livelihoods. Unfortunately, the human body cannot tell the difference between the two, which means we often experience the same physiological reaction to the experience of being stuck in traffic and late for a meeting with the boss as we do when we face a life-and-death situation.

Part of the reason for this is simple: Through most of our existence, humans have faced absolute stressors, situations in which our lives really were at risk. Our bodies adapted to these fears by developing biological mechanisms that would give us the best chance of surviving.

"In prehistoric times," said Dr. Lupien,

> we had to kill the mammoth in order to feed the tribe. So we were forced to come face to face with the mammoth, and that was surely an absolute stressor. You could be killed facing such a beast. Your body wants to survive. Part of you wants to run away from the beast, and another part wants to eat. Your brain knows this, it sees the danger, and therefore signals a stress response.

The biology of that response is now well understood. At the recognition of danger, the hypothalamus, an endocrine organ located in the brain, releases a substance called corticotropin-releasing hormone (CRH). The CRH triggers another gland, the pituitary, also located in the brain, to secrete a second hormone called adrenocorticotropin (ACTH).

ACTH travels in the bloodstream to the adrenal glands, located above your kidneys, and signals them to release adrenaline and a family of stress hormones. The first of these are known as *glucocorticoids* (the most widely known of which is cortisol); the second are known as *catecholamines* (specifically epinephrine and norepinephrine). These substances combine to increase heart rate, respiration, and smooth muscle function. At the same time, blood sugars and fats that are stored in the body are released into the bloodstream so that they can be utilized for energy. In the face of rising glucose and blood fats, insulin levels spike to open up cells to the abundance of fuel that's suddenly available.

This highly potent cocktail of hormones, blood fats, glucose, and insulin triggers the well-known "fight or flight" response, which is part of our survival instinct. Suddenly, you can now run faster, jump higher, lift heavier objects, and fight for your life.

"The beauty of the system is that when you faced the mammoth, or some other threat to your life, your body responded by giving you the energy you needed to fight or flee," says Dr. Lupien.

"Because the human body does not make a distinction between an absolute stressor or a relative stressor," Dr. Lupien continues, "all the same biochemical events that happen when we face the mammoth also happen when you are sitting in your car late for a meeting." Except one, and it's an important one.

"The difference is that when you face a mammoth, you are going to need a lot of energy, and you're going to expend a lot of energy," she points out. That means that all that glucose and all those triglycerides that are released into the bloodstream in the face of a threat are now going be burned as fuel. The fight or the flight is going to utilize all the glucose that your body has suddenly made available to you. When the fight or flight is over, you're going to be hungry for food, because you just expended all your energy reserves.

"But when you're sitting at your desk or in your car and experiencing stress, that glucose and fat are suddenly available in your bloodstream are not going to be burned as fuel," said Dr. Lupien. "Instead, they're going to cause your insulin levels to rise. You may burn a little, but the rest you're going to store as fat." This is the first step in a process in which stress actually increases our weight.

For the person experiencing stress while sitting in his car, the increased levels of glucose and blood fats are also going to drive up cholesterol levels, which are going to have an adverse effect on the heart and arteries.

As if all of this were not enough, another survival mechanism kicks into gear, much to the modern person's detriment. His brain believes that he just faced the mammoth, or the saber-toothed tiger, and consequently has expended all his energy. That means that the brain is going to cause him to think he's hungry, which means he's going to eat more, even though he's got an overabundance of fuel that he'll have to store in his tissues as fat.

"The same hormones that combine to give you energy, the glucocorticoids, have this strange property of going back to the brain and telling the brain that you've just expended energy and you need to eat," Dr. Lupien says. "The glucocorticoids are steroids and capable of crossing the blood-brain barrier within minutes of experiencing stress. Once the stressor has passed, they signal the brain that energy has been burned and must be replaced."

This is one of the reasons why people eat so much when they are under chronic stress, which is the case for so many of us today. Our bodies believe that we have been foraging for food, or facing down some hostile creature that had to be killed in order to survive.

We also eat to relieve the tension that is stored in our muscles as a consequence of the stressor. A study done by Tanja C. Adam and Elissa S. Epel, published in *Physiology and Behavior* (July 2007) reported that, "A subgroup, possibly around 30 percent, decreases food intake and loses weight during or after stress, while most individuals increase their food intake during stress." Adam and Epel report that most people not only increase food intake, but choose foods that are especially dense in calories. For most Westerners, that means choosing processed foods, such as pastries, bagels, chips, or bread, or choosing foods that are rich in fat, such as ice cream, chocolate, cheese, and other dairy products. "The combination of high cortisol, dense calories, and consequently high insulin contributes to the visceral fat distribution," Adam and Epel report. By visceral fat, they mean the fat that's around your waist.

EASILY ACCESSIBLE FAT

We needed calories when we faced the wooly mammoth, but we also needed them in a place where they could be rapidly mobilized and made available to us in seconds. Evolution found just the place for those fatty calories—your belly.

"The body doesn't know about our ideas of beauty or health," Dr. Lupien says. "On the contrary, it says, 'Listen, you have a lot of mammoths in your life—that's why you're always in the stress response.' You need a lot of energy to fight them off, which means you're going to have to eat a lot and store as many calories as you can."

Whenever you are under chronic stress, your brain will create regular bouts of hunger, even when your body has plenty of stored energy. And it will store those excess calories on your belly as a form of rapidly available, emergency energy. The consequence of these two survival mechanisms—increased hunger and accumulation of calories around your waist—is overweight and potential obesity.

As Dr. Lupien puts it, "The body says 'I figured out that if I store the glucose and fat in my abdomen, then I can use it faster.' This is why we, in the field of stress research, see abdominal obesity as a good marker for chronic stress. Other factors change, as well.

Heart rate is definitely going to increase. So, too, does cholesterol."

The sudden availability of blood fats is going to drive up cholesterol levels. But there's another reason cholesterol goes up. The body needs cholesterol to make hormones, including stress hormones, which means that the more stress the body experiences, the more it will need cholesterol in order to make stress hormones. "So if your body needs a lot of stress hormone, you will need to eat foods that increase your cholesterol levels," says Dr. Lupien.

As weight, triglycerides, cholesterol, and insulin levels rise, so too does inflammation. Now you have the foundation for a whole host of serious illnesses, including diabetes, heart disease, and many forms of cancer.

"There are many studies that show that an increase in glucocorticoids will lead to an increase in insulin, and insulin resistance, which will then lead to an increase in type 2 diabetes," Dr. Lupien says.

FACING THE BOSS

One of the problems we face in the twenty-first century is clearly identifying what constitutes an actual threat—in other words, a truly stressful situation—versus a situation that only appears to be threatening, but really isn't. In short, we haven't figured out as yet when to be stressed out and when to relax. Some of this is due to our biology, and some of it is our failure to adapt.

Hans Selye, the pioneer Canadian stress researcher, first identified the stress response in 1936. Selye spent most of his time researching physical reactions to stress, such as the effects of heat and cold on the body and nervous system. Based on his research, Selye extrapolated that any stressful situation could cause a stress response.

But in 1968, psychologist John Mason, PhD, came along and questioned Selye's theory. He said that the body can adapt to stress, especially when a stressful situation is repeated over time. Mason did a series of experiments in which he monitored the stress hormones released by people in a wide variety of stressful situations. Among his subjects were a group of people who parachuted out of airplanes. Mason studied both men and women who jumped for the first time, as well as instructors who had made such jumps dozens of times.

Mason found that right before they went into the airplane, the first-time jumpers experienced acute escalations in stress hormones. Mason thus concluded that jumping from airplanes is, indeed, highly stressful. But then he found something interesting. The trainers' stress levels remained normal when they got into the plane and even made their jumps. For them, jumping out of an airplane was routine. Not only was it routine, but it didn't represent a significant threat to the trainers. In other words, there was no reason to be afraid, as far as they were concerned.

"The first-time jumpers didn't know what to expect," says Dr. Lupien. "For them, this was a frightening experience. Moreover, they didn't feel in control of the situation. The trainers, on the other hand, did know what to expect. They didn't feel it was especially dangerous, and they were in control." From these experiments, Mason came up with a set of four criteria that formed the foundation for a stressful event. All four characteristics do not have to be met,

Dr. Lupien says, but the more of them that are met, the more stressful the situation is.

Those four characteristics are as follows:

1. Novelty. The situation must be new to the person, and therefore foreign. The less we know how to behave in situations, the more stressful they are.
2. Unpredictability. The outcome of the event must be unpredictable. When something is at risk and we are uncertain as to how the situation will unfold, the more stressful it is.
3. Threat. Something we value must be at risk to be stressful. When a situation poses a threat to our lives, our livelihoods, or our identity, it is considered stressful. It's important to remember that identity can include our status and our ego identification with the outcome of a project or situation. The person who is known for always being on time can experience a great deal of stress if he is stuck in traffic.
4. Sense of no control. Situations that pose a risk and are out of our control are inherently stressful. And the greater the risk, and the more out of control the situation seems, the more stressful they are.

Using the first letter in each of the four criteria, Dr. Mason coined the acronym NUTS as the basis for interpreting whether or not a situation was stressful.

As Dr. Lupien points out, we face situations every day that we interpret as a threat to our identities or our livelihoods, which means most of us are dealing with NUTS on a daily basis. That is especially the case at work, where stressful situations seem to arise on a daily basis. According to the American Institute of Stress, fully 80 percent of American workers say that they feel stressed on their jobs, and nearly half say that they need help coping with stress. Sixty-two percent of workers say that they routinely end the workday with work-related neck pain, and 34 percent say that stress disrupts their ability to sleep at night.

"Our body doesn't know that it's 2007," says Dr. Lupien. "Our body does not make a difference between an absolute stressor and a relative stressor. This means your brain will not make a distinction between a mammoth and Sarah, the boss at work, who stresses you out every day."

STRESS, INSULIN, AND CANCER

Lee Roy Morgan, MD, PhD, is the retired head of the pharmacology department at Louisiana State University Medical Center in New Orleans. He has also worked closely with the National Institutes of Health to develop an array of pharmaceutical agents to treat disease, including drugs to treat cancer. In addition to being a long-time researcher at LSU, Dr. Morgan is a general practitioner, seeing patients for more than thirty years; he knows a lot about factors in health and disease that don't come in textbooks. He has observed firsthand the relationship of stress and cancer. As stress raises insulin levels, it also causes a sharp increase in insulin-like growth factor (IGF-1), which in turn promotes the life of malignant cells and tumors.

"When a person experiences negative stress, the body causes a breakdown in fat and carbohydrate stores, which causes glucose levels to spike and insulin levels to go up," Dr. Morgan says. "Prolonged stress leads to chronically high insulin and IGF-1 levels, which in turn makes a person vulnerable to cancer."

Dr. Morgan also takes into account the fact that when people are under stress, their diets and exercise habits tend to change. Very often, more fat, processed foods, and alcohol are consumed, all of which increase insulin and IGF-1 levels.

"I have seen that very stressful events, such as divorce, bankruptcy, job loss, or the sickness or loss of a loved one, cause a dramatic change in blood chemistry," Dr. Morgan says. "Then eighteen months to two years later, a person is diagnosed with cancer."

Dr. Morgan, who has spent much of his professional life living in New Orleans, expresses great concern over the residents of New Orleans in the aftermath of Hurricane Katrina. He's concerned that the devastation from the hurricane, and the many broken lives it has left behind, may bring on waves of illness among the residents. "Unless the people of this city get help, we may see waves of illness strike the people," he said. "I hope that is not the case, but I'm concerned. This has been one of the most stressful events in our history—a whole city wiped out—and the stress is going to hit the people hard."

HOW TO COPE WITH STRESS

If stress elevates important blood constituents, and forms the conditions for major illness, the best way to combat stress is to burn fuel. We must, in effect, recreate the reaction our ancient ancestors had to stressors themselves. They burned energy when they faced the wooly mammoth. We have to do the same when we face the stressors of modern life.

Once we begin exercising, the first reserves of fat that we will burn will be in our muscles, our livers, and in our stomachs. Stomach fat is quickly mobilized and made available to our cells whenever our energy levels fall, especially when we are using our muscles in any form of exertion. The body is going to surrender that stored energy very rapidly during exercise.

"Whenever I am under stress, I run," Dr. Lupien said. "The reason is simple. I know my body is going to start storing calories as fat, and that's going to have a big impact on my health. So I have to increase my exercise to burn off the calories that my body is going to accumulate. In effect, I have to do something physical that would burn calories as if I were fighting the mammoth. So whenever my neighbors see me running, they know I'm under stress."

A half-hour of vigorous exercise per day is all it takes to burn the fat that has accumulated on the body, and particularly around the middle. Perhaps the best program for exercise is to combine some form of vigorous exercise that you do a few times a week, with a more gentle form, such as a half-hour a day of walking. If you do not have a half hour per day, do three ten-minute walks. The research shows that three ten-minute walks have an accumulating effect that amounts to that thirty-minute walk.

The best way to get some form of vigorous exercise is to find a game or a practice that you really enjoy. Consider taking up tennis, racquetball, or volleyball; perform a martial art; do aerobic or ballroom dancing, swing, or tango; run on a treadmill; or do some other physical activity that you enjoy, and engage in it at least three times per week. Yoga is typically thought of as gentle exercise, but anyone who does yoga regularly knows it's a workout. Try doing some yoga three to five times a week, and couple it with a daily walk. You'll find your conditioning will improve rapidly.

In addition to that walk and an enjoyable, vigorous practice, be active every day. Walk up the steps to your office, or take short walks from your car to your office. Get your heart rate up, even for a few minutes, to improve circulation, engage your muscles, and move your body.

Exercise alone can lower insulin levels, build muscle, and burn fat. And in the process, it can protect you from the range of serious illnesses that arise from high stress and high insulin.

On the other hand, serious consequences result if changes in behavior—especially exercise and diet—do not occur in the face of chronic stress. Dr. Lupien points out that chronic stress, along with chronic elevations in insulin, can lead to various kinds of adaptation, or what scientists refer to as *dysregulation*, including in the brain. Dysregulation of brain function that is sustained over time can lead to neurological disorders, including Alzheimer's.

Very few people think of Alzheimer's disease as having anything to do with insulin, but researchers are now discovering that even this terrible disease may well be the consequence of insulin resistance.

· 8 ·

Alzheimer's, Memory Loss,
and Dementia

Few aspects of aging are more terrifying than the specter of having your mind swallowed whole by the darkness that is Alzheimer's disease. Anyone who has witnessed a loved one's slow withdrawal into that lost and unreachable realm knows. Alzheimer's is a mind robber. Gradually, inexorably, it steals your memory and your sense of self until all of those whom you have loved, and all who have loved you, become part of a parade of passing strangers. Past, present, and future are a blur. The memories and relationships that define you as a unique person collapse and disappear in the dim mists of dementia.

Alzheimer's disease is a neurological disorder that causes the slow, progressive loss of memory. It is accompanied by confusion, withdrawal from social contact, gradual loss of speech, emotional agitation, uncontrolled muscle movement, incontinence, and often hallucinations. The illness can last as long as twenty-five years, but usually causes death within eight to ten years of onset. It was originally diagnosed by German physician Alois Alzheimer, who recognized two abnormal characteristics in the brains of people who were afflicted with the disease—the presence of amyloid plaques (essentially scar tissue in the brain) and the twisting of microtubules, also known as *neurofibrillary tangles,* which, in health, allow nutrients to flow within nerve cells or neurons. When these tiny tubules become damaged or twisted, the flow of nutrients ceases and the cells die. Great swaths of gray matter are lost in the Alzheimer brain, along with the brain's ability to produce adequate quantities of a chemical neurotransmitter known as acetylcholine, which is essential to experiencing memory.

These symptoms, which characterize Alzheimer's disease, contrast with the more common form of dementia, which usually arises when the brain is deprived of oxygen. In common dementia, atherosclerosis has caused the diminution of blood flow to crucial areas of the brain, causing brain dysfunction and memory loss. Standard dementia is not associated with the extensive swaths of amyloid plaques and neurofibrillary tangles that are seen in Alzheimer's disease.

Alzheimer's disease currently afflicts some 4.5 million Americans, or one in ten over the age of sixty-five. Nearly half of all Americans eighty-five and older have Alzheimer's.

The number of people with Alzheimer's disease is now exploding. In the 1980s alone, incidence of Alzheimer's rose 1,000 percent. Physicians are quick to point out that part of that increase is due to heightened awareness—doctors are more likely to label dementia as Alzheimer's today. Nevertheless, leading researchers in the field point out that even when increased awareness is taken into account, the numbers of people showing up with Alzheimer's is rising dramatically. Health experts predict that by the year 2050, more than fourteen million Americans will suffer from Alzheimer's. Like so many other rising illnesses—metabolic syndrome and diabetes, for example—this one poses a tremendous threat to our health care system.

One of the many aspects of Alzheimer's that make it so frightening is that researchers do not understand how it develops. While different theories abound, many scientists would say that the cause of Alzheimer's is unknown. Complicating the picture is the fact that genetic research has revealed that only 15 to 25 percent of all Alzheimer's cases are considered purely genetic in origin—that is, the consequence of inherited traits passed down from parents and ancestors. But new and persuasive clues have been mounting, and due to the work of leading scientists, a clear picture of the causes of Alzheimer's has started to emerge.

INSULIN'S ROLE IN THE BRAIN

Over the past few years, it has become clear that insulin plays a profound role in brain function. In addition to regulating appetite, it is now appreciated that insulin signaling is crucial for learning, memory, behavior, and survival of brain cells. Insulin activates critical brain neurotransmitters, including dopamine and acetylcholine, and insulin resistance is linked to diminished levels of dopamine and acetylcholine, leading to addiction, obesity, ADHD, and Alzheimer's disease.

ALZHEIMER'S DISEASE—
A THIRD FORM OF DIABETES

Alzheimer's, many scientists now believe, is a form of diabetes of the brain. Indeed, one of the world's leading Alzheimer's researchers, Suzanne de la Monte, MD, MPH, of Brown University's Alpert Medical School, is now referring to Alzheimer's disease as "type 3 diabetes"—meaning a type of diabetes that destroys brain cells and leads to dementia.

"In Alzheimer's disease, brain cells cannot respond to insulin appropriately," Dr. de la Monte told us in an interview. "Neurons, like all other cells, require insulin to produce ATP (adenosine triphosphate, the fuel used by cells). If they cannot respond to insulin, then normal energy production, metabolism, and cell signaling doesn't happen, and among the things you get is low production of acetylcholine."

This revelation has opened doors to new and possibly effective therapeutic avenues. Researchers have found that inhaled insulin significantly improved memory in normal elderly people. Inhaled insulin is now being considered as a potential treatment for Alzheimer's disease.

Not only are these revelations leading to new forms of treatment, but scientists are recognizing new approaches to prevention. Clearly, prevention begins by recognizing the need to keep insulin levels under control, and by avoiding metabolic syndrome and diabetes.

People with diabetes are twice as likely to develop Alzheimer's as nondiabetics. The same amyloid plaques that build up in the brains of Alzheimer's victims appear in the pancreases of diabetics. Moreover, researchers say when metabolic syndrome is added to the picture—that is, overweight, high blood pressure, high glucose, and high insulin levels—the risk of Alzheimer's skyrockets.

A study done by Rachel A. Whitmer, PhD, and her colleagues at Kaiser Permanente in Oakland, California, followed more than 22,000 patients for eight years. The study participants who developed full-blown diabetes had the highest risk of Alzheimer's. In fact, those with the highest blood sugar levels had an 83 percent greater risk of contracting Alzheimer's than those whose blood sugar levels remained normal.

Insulin levels are directly related to weight. As insulin rises, so, too, does weight gain. It's for this reason that the overwhelming majority of people with type 2 diabetes are overweight. Following this strong connection, Dr. Whitmer did another study in which she followed 10,276 men and women for seven years. As she and her colleagues found, those people who gained the most weight in middle age had the greatest risk of developing Alzheimer's disease. Of those who became overweight in middle age, 35 percent developed Alzheimer's later in life. Of those who became obese, 74 percent developed Alzheimer's.

Not only are overweight and obesity indicators of rising insulin levels, but they are also associated with high blood pressure and high cholesterol—in short, metabolic syndrome, which researchers have found dramatically raises the risk of contracting Alzheimer's disease. One study found that people who are overweight and borderline diabetics—in essence, those who suffer from metabolic syndrome—were 70 percent more likely to get Alzheimer's than lean nondiabetics.

There are forty-one million Americans with metabolic syndrome, all of whom are at increased risk of contracting Alzheimer's. Not all of them will get Alzheimer's, of course—in large part because many will die from some other insulin-related illness such as heart disease, cancer, stroke, or from other complications stemming from diabetes.

TURNING NEURONS INTO SCAR TISSUE

Dr. de la Monte has been exploring the link between brain levels of insulin and Alzheimer's disease for much of the past decade. A neuropathologist and associate professor of pathology and medicine at Brown, Dr. de la Monte is one of the pioneers in revealing the link between insulin resistance and Alzheimer's. Indeed, her research won her the first-ever Alzheimer Award in 2000 for making the year's outstanding contribution to our understanding of the disease.

Among the questions that have baffled researchers are: Why do the brains of those who suffer from this illness accumulate a toxic protein, known as *beta amyloid*? All human brains produce this protein, but people with Alzheimer's disease do not clear the protein from the brain. Instead, it accumulates and eventually forms amyloid plaques, which disrupt neuron signaling and eventually cut off production of acetylcholine.

Another question is: Why do the neurons in Alzheimer's patients become twisted, or tangled up, into these convoluted masses of inert tissue?

In her search for answers, Dr. de la Monte and her colleagues examined the brains of forty-five deceased people who suffered from Alzheimer's disease and compared them to the post-mortem brains of people who had not suffered from the illness. What the researchers found was startling. The Alzheimer brains showed significantly fewer insulin receptors on their neurons, indicating that insulin could not be taken effectively into cells. Without insulin, cells die, but not before undergoing dramatic and destructive changes.

"Those with the most advanced Alzheimer's disease had nearly 80 percent fewer insulin receptors than normal brains," says Dr. de la Monte. The researchers also discovered that as insulin levels in the neurons fell, neurons died and Alzheimer's disease progressed.

Insulin wasn't the only essential substance that was lowered inside of neurons. So, too, was insulin-like growth factor, IGF-1. Contrary to what goes on in cancer, where too much IGF-1 can stimulate tumor growth, the human brain requires IGF-1 in order to support neuron function. Not only does IGF-1 stimulate cell growth, but in the brain it makes neuronal connections more complex, thus allowing for more complex forms of thought to take place. Growth factors are part of the reason human brains are capable of learning and thinking creatively.

However, without adequate numbers of insulin receptors on the neurons, brain cells cannot absorb adequate quantities of insulin and glucose. Nor can they be stimulated by IGF-1. Declines in insulin, glucose, and growth factors cause gradual reduction in neuron function and eventually cell death. People with Alzheimer's are losing brain cells—in effect, their brains are shrinking—and with such losses go memory and other cerebral functions.

Scientists are trying to understand why this brain loss occurs. In fact, although insulin isn't stimulating cells to absorb glucose, it is present in the brain, at least in the early stages of Alzheimer's disease. The insulin is not being absorbed by cells as it would in a normally functioning brain. In fact, in people with Alzheimer's, insulin is accumulating in the blood and tissue of the brain. Because high levels of insulin are toxic, the brain recognizes the excess insulin as a threat and utilizes a particular protein, called insulin-degrading enzyme (IDE), to clear the insulin from the blood supply.

The problem is that IDE is also used to clear beta amyloid—the protein that leads to the creation of amyloid plaques, which in turn disrupt brain function. In effect, the excess insulin competes with beta amyloid for IDE. Unfortunately, the insulin wins—meaning it robs the brain of the IDE it would otherwise use to clear beta amyloid.

That means that the more insulin in the blood, the less IDE there is for the brain to clear the beta amyloid protein. As beta amyloid accumulates, it creates plaques and scarring of brain tissue, which leads to the loss of acetylcholine, loss of memory, and cell death.

NEURON TANGLES

The accumulation of beta amyloid is not the only destructive process that leads to Alzheimer's, however. There is also the creation of those twists and tangles that destroy the microtubule canals within neurons. Again, insulin resistance sets off a domino effect of damage of kinases within cells that eventually leads to the tangling of neurons.

In a healthy brain, stable insulin levels raise a kinase within the cell called Akt. Akt, in turn, inhibits another kinase, found downstream from Akt, which is called GSK-3. In effect, Akt is a good cop to GSK-3, which can get out of hand if not restrained. Unfortunately, in insulin resistance, Akt levels drop and GSK-3 rises. In effect, the police force is weakened and the GSK-3 gang gets stronger and goes wild. The elevated GSK-3 levels overstimulate a protein known as *tau*, which is when damage to cells begins to happen.

Tau is the engineer of the microtubules inside your neurons. It helps grow and maintain these canals in which nutrients flow. But when GSK-3 levels rise, they overstimulate tau, which causes the protein to misbehave. Tau is overstimulated, making it hyperactive and chaotic. The result is that tau turns those beautiful and orderly tubules into a tangle of weaves and meshes that destroy neurons, which then die and cause the loss of brain function.

Ideally, GSK-3 should be under the control of Akt, which keeps the kinase relatively quiescent. In that state, GSK-3 gently supports tau. But in insulin resistance, both kinases become disrupted and all that orderly plumbing in the brain is turned into a jumble of disorganization that is reflected in brain dysfunction.

Stated simply, insulin signaling plays an essential role in the survival of brain cells. In insulin-resistant brains, the brain forms amyloid plaques and tau proteins, the two destructive substances that form the basis for Alzheimer's disease.

THE ROLE OF INFLAMMATION

As we said in chapter 5, insulin resistance doesn't exist without its partner in crime, inflammation. This destructive duo is involved in the disruption of brain chemistry as well.

High insulin results in high levels of beta amyloid. As it accumulates, beta amyloid begins to decay or break down, and in the process releases free radicals. These highly reactive oxygen molecules, in turn, cause the breakdown of cells, eventually destroying many neurons. Your immune system recognizes the problem and sends in macrophages to repair the damage. But in trying to restore health, the immune cells release cytokines—including interleukin-6—that are highly inflammatory. These chemical messengers call forth armies of additional immune cells, which release more free radicals and more cytokines. As crowds of immune cells gather, more inflammation occurs in the area, cutting off oxygen flow to cells and deforming and destroying more neurons.

Dr. de la Monte says that inflammation is occurring at the early stages of Alzheimer's, but researchers still don't fully understand all the sources of that inflammation. "Some kind of proinflammatory response is occurring as a consequence of the presence of macrophages and cytokines," Dr. de la Monte says, "but we don't fully understand the cause of the inflammation. The inflammation that's taking place in the brain is extremely subtle. If I hadn't measured it, I would not have seen it. But inflammation plays a critical role." Indeed, inflammation is part of the constellation of factors in the brain that are killing brain cells.

The fact that inflammation is occurring at the early stages of the illness gives scientists some hope for an effective treatment. "Inflammation is occurring in diabetes, as with many other degenerative diseases," Dr. de la Monte says. "If you suppress it in diabetes, you can ameliorate the disorder. In the brain, you have inflammatory responses going on and they are taking place early on, so that if we could detect and reduce the inflammation, we might be better able to control the illness."

INFLAMMATION, VASCULAR DISEASE, AND DEMENTIA

By killing neurons, inflammation can dramatically reduce brain function and acetylcholine production. But it also can trigger nascent Alzheimer's, or accelerate the early stages of the disease by reducing the blood and oxygen flow to the brain.

This is a new understanding of Alzheimer's—that it is often accompanied, and made worse, by atherosclerosis (vascular disease) in the vessels that bring blood and oxygen to the brain.

Inflammation causes atherosclerosis in the carotid arteries, located in the neck, that bring blood flow to the brain. It is also the basis for high blood pressure that injures arteries as well. High blood cholesterol and high blood pressure combine to trigger an immune reaction—inflammation—in the tissues of arteries and lead to the creation of artery plaques. Once those plaques grow large enough, they can block blood and oxygen supply to the brain. The result is impaired brain function, neuronal cell death, and eventually dementia.

"Vascular disease is a contributing factor in the creation of Alzheimer's," says Dr. de la Monte. "When you look at the brains of people with Alzheimer's disease, what you find is that about 40 percent of them have Alzheimer's disease and vascular disease," said Dr. de la Monte. "They really have two kinds of dementia going on at the same time: Alzheimer's disease and what is called vascular dementia."

For those who may be in jeopardy of developing Alzheimer's, vascular disease only increases the danger. "If you have a low level of Alzheimer's and you have bad vessel disease, it can bring on the illness, or make it worse," said Dr. de la Monte.

Numerous studies have corroborated Dr. de la Monte's statement. A five-year study published in *The Journal of the American Medical Association* (November 10, 2004) that followed 2,632 men and women, all in their seventies, and all with metabolic syndrome, found that those with the highest levels of inflammation had the highest rates of dementia.

In a study published in *Neurobiology of Aging* (December 2005), researchers concluded, "Our data suggest that excessive insulin invokes synchronous increases in levels of Abeta [beta amyloid plaques] and inflammatory agents, effects that are exacerbated by age and obesity. This constellation of events may have deleterious effects on memory." Other studies have resulted in similar findings.

These links between inflammation and disease explain why people with metabolic syndrome are so much at risk for Alzheimer's disease and other forms of dementia. They have all the markers for increased risk of Alzheimer's, including high insulin, overweight, high blood pressure, and high cholesterol—all of which combine to decrease blood and oxygen to the brain and trigger the onset of Alzheimer's disease.

There is a silver lining. By recognizing that insulin resistance, inflammation, and vascular disease all play a role in the onset of Alzheimer's, doctors are offered an array of new approaches to prevent and treat the illness.

NEW HOPE FOR ALZHEIMER'S

One of the first issues researchers are encouraging people to recognize is that insulin resistance and overweight must be avoided at all costs. "Obesity in middle age increases the risk of future dementia," Dr. Whitmer concluded. She told *The New York Times* (July 17, 2006) that people must control their blood sugar levels throughout life, but this becomes especially important as we approach old age.

"Tight control is important for the whole life span," Dr. Whitmer said. "The older you are, the more likely you are to get dementia." This means, of course, that diets rich in calories and saturated fat must be avoided. Processed and fatty foods drive up insulin levels and lead to weight gain, insulin resistance, and type 2 diabetes. They also lead to atherosclerosis and artery disease, thus increasing the odds of Alzheimer's.

Dr. Whitmer offered a stark warning if such advice isn't heeded. "With the whole diabetes epidemic, we're seeing much more type 2, so are we going to see even more Alzheimer's than we thought we would see? If we continue in this direction, it's a little bit frightening."

Keeping insulin levels within healthy ranges is essential. A diet rich in unprocessed plant foods and low-fat animal foods, especially fish, not only will keep your insulin and weight down, but it will also protect your arteries, and thus keep blood and oxygen flowing to your brain.

Researchers have noted for many years that Japanese people living in Japan have far lower rates of Alzheimer's and dementia than Japanese who come to the United States and adopt an American way of eating. Japanese living in Japan eat diets that are rich in grains, vegetables, and fish, while those living in America eat a diet that's far richer in calories and animal foods, and thus saturated fat. Other differences in disease patterns between Westerners and Asians—especially in breast, prostate, and colon cancers—are consistent with this same finding.

This same trend has been found in Africans versus African Americans—and not coincidentally, the latter have far higher rates of Alzheimer's. Rates of Alzheimer's vary greatly around the world and there is a probable link to the predominant diet in each area. Researchers analyzed Alzheimer rates and dietary patterns in twelve different countries and concluded that, "Diet, dietary fat, and to a lesser extent, total energy (caloric intake) were found to be significant risk factors for the development of AD . . . , while fish consumption" significantly reduced the risk. Writing in the *Journal of Alzheimer's Disease* (June 2002), the researchers also pointed out that diets rich in whole grains and vegetables also lowered the risk of the disease.

In a study entitled "Mediterranean Diet and Cognitive Decline," published in *Public Health Nutrition* (October 2004), researchers found that the standard Mediterranean diet—rich in complex carbohydrates from grains and vegetables, monounsaturated fats from olive oil, and red wine—was associated with much lower rates of age-related cognitive decline (ARCD) or dementia. They found that consumption of olive oil appeared to be particularly protective. "It cannot be excluded that the positive effect of dietary habits on cognitive functioning among healthy elderly subjects could be due in part to the antioxidant compounds of olive oil," wrote the researchers. Antioxidants reduce the rate of oxidation and lower inflammation. Virtually all plant foods are rich in antioxidants, as are high-quality plant oils such as olive oil.

In addition to diet, the activity that is most protective of your arteries is exercise. Exercise alone will lower insulin levels, create greater insulin sensitivity in cells, lower blood pressure, and lower inflammation. It also raises HDL cholesterol, which protects the arteries throughout the body. Alzheimer researcher Weili Xu, MD, points out that exercise and diet combined can reverse borderline diabetes and may help prevent dementia.

That was the conclusion of a study examining 1,740 healthy adults, sixty-five years and older, and published in the *Annals of Internal Medicine* (January 17, 2006). The researchers found that those people who exercised at least three times per week were far less likely to develop any form of dementia, including Alzheimer's disease, than those who exercised less frequently, or not at all.

More and more researchers are looking at lifestyle factors as the underlying cause of Alzheimer's disease. Noting that only a small fraction of Alzheimer's arises purely from genetic reasons, scientists are looking increasingly at daily diet and exercise patterns as perhaps the true underlying cause of the disease. As the researchers on the Mediterranean diet concluded, "the prevalence of AD is more strongly influenced by diet and nutrition, environment and/or lifestyle than by genetics."

Such a revelation cuts both ways. While it reveals potential future health risks, especially if we persist in following a diet and lifestyle that supports insulin resistance, overweight, and diabetes, it also offers ways to protect ourselves and our loved ones from the illness.

Treating insulin resistance and its related disorders is not the only approach we can take, however. There are other steps that may protect us, as well.

EXERCISE YOUR MIND

Studies have shown that those who keep learning well into their senior years have much lower rates of Alzheimer's disease.

"There's a lot of ways to look at this phenomenon," says Richard S. Jope, PhD, professor of psychiatry and behavioral neurobiology at the University of Alabama School of Medicine.

"When you get Alzheimer's disease, you lose a lot of neurons before you experience any cognitive deficit," he said. "So people who read a lot may be the ones who started out in life with more neurons—they have a big surplus—so that they can lose a lot of neurons before they experience any sort of impairment. That's one way of looking at it."

On other hand, living a more intellectually challenging and adventurous life may be inherently good for the brain. "Another way of looking at things is to see the brain as a muscle," says Dr. Jope. "And like any muscle, the same rules apply. Use it or lose it." In fact, scientists have found that learning stimulates brain cells to produce more growth factors, such as IGF-1, which sustain neurons and with them our ability to learn, to think complex thoughts, and to retrieve memories.

Numerous studies have supported this perspective. Scientists have found that a supportive environment, with ample stimulation and regular demands for learning new skills, may protect the brain from premature cell death.

A study published in *Nature Medicine* (April 1999) showed that animals placed in environments that were both supportive and stimulating experienced much lower rates of cell apoptosis within the brain than animals that were made to live in isolation. The researchers concluded that "a complex, enriched environment has important effects on brain function, by providing resilience to . . . insults [to brain tissue] as well as stimulating new cell birth and preventing cell death."

Similar findings have been shown in human research as well. Those who achieve higher levels of education, and go on learning new skills well into their later years, have far lower rates of Alzheimer's and other forms of dementia.

Clearly, humans need to be challenged and to grow in order to feel alive. Such basic needs, born of tens of thousands of years of experience, may well be woven into our DNA. Among the lessons of Alzheimer's may be that without external stimulation and a pressing need to learn and adapt, the human brain atrophies and eventually dies. Evidence of this fact has turned up throughout human history.

In their book *A General Theory of Love* (Random House, 2000), authors Thomas Lewis, MD, Fari Amini, MD, and Richard Lannon, MD, point to the experience of Frederick II, a thirteenth-century Italian king who instructed his nurses and staff to avoid all forms of communication with his children. The king believed that if he kept his children isolated from all forms of speech, they would spontaneously begin speaking the innate language of humans, which the king assumed would be either Hebrew, Greek, Latin, Arabic, or Italian. Unfortunately, all his children died before they spoke a word. A Franciscan monk who observed the king's experiment later noted that the children needed communication of all sorts in order to develop normally and stay alive.

Life is expressed by our need to learn, to share our inner thoughts and feelings, to experience connection with others, and to constantly grow from our experiences. Clearly, such adventures in learning are among the fundamental needs that keep us healthy and alive. When it comes to Alzheimer's disease, many other factors must be taken into account as well. Among them are a healthy way of eating, engaging in physical activity, and maintaining a healthy weight. No doubt, researchers will soon discover other important protective behaviors. What we have learned to date gives us a clear direction, and may be enough to protect ourselves, and those we love, from the multiple scourges that torment the body and destroy the mind, before they snuff out our lives.

· 9 ·

Children at Risk

Adam, an eleven-year-old in the fifth grade, has brown hair, freckles, and is eighteen pounds overweight. His parents refer to him as "stocky," but his physique clearly foretells the future: Unless dramatic changes occur, he will battle weight issues for the rest of his life. That may be the lesser of his problems. As he sits at his desk at school, Adam is intensely restless and has great difficulty giving his attention to his school work for longer than thirty seconds. He fidgets with his pencil, looks over at his neighbor to his right, looks back at his teacher, and then to his neighbor on his left. His feet bounce up and down on the floor. He reaches for a piece of paper in his notebook and starts drawing impulsively on the paper. His expression remains detached and impassive, even when he draws a large X over the picture he has made. He raises his hand and asks his teacher if he can go to the bathroom. Permission is denied. He seems unaffected by his teacher's response, as if her words were never spoken. Instead, he continues to look around the room, apparently searching for something to engage his attention for longer than twenty seconds. Adam suffers from attention deficit hyperactivity disorder (ADHD), and this is one of his better days.

William was nineteen years old when he started to believe that the CIA was monitoring and directing his thoughts. At twenty-one, he began to hear voices in his head on a daily basis. His paranoid delusions worsened and he was soon diagnosed with schizophrenia. Now twenty-six, William has been on every drug available, including a pharmaceutical called clozapine, which his doctors admit has contributed to a significant increase in weight. William is not only overweight, but he has metabolic syndrome that very likely will become type 2 diabetes within the decade. Meanwhile, his symptoms continue to haunt him. He bounces around between small jobs at convenience stores and video rental outlets and receives state-sponsored disability.

Nancy, thirteen years old, suffers from pediatric bipolar disorder, often referred to as manic depression. She experiences wild swings in mood and energy levels, going from deep states of depression, disinterest in her surroundings, and lethargy, to sudden mania, hyperactive behavior, and delusions of grandeur. At times, she believes she can literally jump off the roofs of houses, or leap out of the way of oncoming cars, without any fear of injury. But just as suddenly, she can fall into terrible depression, or irrational fears, or uncontrollable rage. At thirteen years of age, Nancy is coming into puberty and has begun to demonstrate inappropriate sexual behavior. She has already expressed thoughts of suicide to her parents.

Jimmy is nine years old and acutely sensitive to voices and noise.

He is intensely shy and lost in his own internal world. When left to his own devices, he is clearly hyperactive and obsessive. If an adult attempts to speak to him, he refuses to look at the person, and when he does, he stares into the person's mouth, as if it held some kind of secret that has nothing to do with the person's words. When Jimmy speaks, he often repeats phrases over and over again, like a mantra. He seems relieved when his mother holds his hand or touches his body. Jimmy has autism, a brain disorder that is characterized by social withdrawal, inability to communicate feelings and complex thoughts, and intense sensitivity to sensory inputs. All of Jimmy's outward behaviors are a reflection of his brain's anatomy.

When scientists examine the brains of autistic children, they find that certain regions, such as the frontal lobe (the part of the brain that makes higher reasoning possible) and the amygdala (that helps determine threats), are overdeveloped. The normal sculpting of the brain, accomplished in part by apoptosis, has not occurred, causing abnormalities in brain structure and function. For many people with autism, higher reasoning is lost and the perception of threats is exaggerated.

●　●　●

All four of these people suffer from very distinct and different disorders, but their conditions share an underlying set of factors that may play a role in their origin. Researchers do not have all the answers as yet, and much is still shrouded in mystery. But little by little, clues to the origins of mental disorders such as ADHD, manic depression, schizophrenia, and autism are emerging. As they do, a coherent picture is starting to take shape, one that involves a complex array of genetic and environmental factors. And at the heart of this picture is our nemesis, insulin resistance.

Scientists are finding that insulin resistance can spread from the body cells (also known as *somatic cells*) to the cells of the central nervous system and the brain. Once there, they can have a profound effect on brain function, causing—among other conditions—dramatic changes in brain formation and psychological health.

Once insulin resistance takes hold in the brain, it can alter the delicate communication that occurs within neurons and between them, causing dramatic changes in brain function and altering perceptions, thoughts, impulses, moods, and beliefs.

Though still controversial, the theory that insulin resistance is at the bottom of many brain and psychiatric disorders is now finding its way into the highest levels of the medical literature. In an article in *The Journal of the American Medical Association* (October 11, 2006), M. J. Friedrich wrote the following:

> Known best for its role in the body as a regulator of blood glucose levels and fatty acid storage, insulin also acts in the brain to aid memory and thinking. Thus, when insulin regulation is disrupted, as it is in many common medical conditions including obesity and diabetes, the risk for cognitive impairment rises.

That cognitive impairment can take many forms, from Alzheimer's disease to ADHD to schizophrenia to bipolar disorder. Certainly, there are unique genetic factors that make one person susceptible to, say, ADHD, and another to schizophrenia, and still another to autism. However, increasingly scientists are recognizing that insulin resistance can affect different parts of the brain, and thereby alter gene function, which in turn can trigger one or another of these disorders.

In this chapter, we want to report some of the new insights into mental illness, and its links to insulin resistance. Up until a short while ago, these illnesses were inscrutable to researchers and medical doctors alike. But the new evidence holds out the hope that these seemingly disparate illnesses may one day be treated at their common roots. Perhaps even more important, researchers are forming the basis for new methods of prevention. Indeed, these approaches may soon give doctors and parents the practical medical and lifestyle tools to control insulin resistance and thereby protect children from these terrible diseases.

EARLY EVIDENCE

One of the first clues linking impaired insulin function to mental disorders was the realization that so many people with ADHD, schizophrenia, and depression suffer from metabolic syndrome.

One study published in *The Journal of Clinical Psychiatry* (May 2005), showed people with schizophrenia had four times the risk of suffering from metabolic syndrome as healthy adults. Similar results have turned up when scientists examined people suffering from ADHD and bipolar disorder. British researchers studied 215 people who were undergoing treatment for obesity and found that ADHD was "highly prevalent" among obese patients and that the incidence of ADHD was "highest in those with extreme obesity." Of course, having ADHD makes it extremely difficult to adhere to self-help forms of weight-loss treatment, which may explain why obese people have such difficulty following weight-loss programs, the scientists noted (*BMC Psychiatry*, September 13, 2002).

Scientists have noted a correlation between bipolar disorder and metabolic syndrome, and in a review of studies, published in *The Journal of Clinical Psychiatry* (July 2006), researchers concluded that "bipolar disorder and metabolic syndrome share features of hormonal, immunologic, and autonomic nervous system dysregulation."

Increasingly, researchers are finding insulin resistance present in the etiology of autism, as well. Autism is characterized by an abnormal overgrowth of specific regions of the brain including the superior frontal lobe and cerebellum. That overgrowth is followed by abnormally slow brain development. Both of these findings have been established by researchers by measuring head circumference and magnetic resonance imaging (MRI).

Clearly, something has gone wrong in the sculpting of the brain during early development. The gene responsible for shaping the brain during fetal and early life is p53, the guardian of the genome and the trigger of apoptosis. Studies of autistic children by S. H. Fatemi and M. Araghi-Niknam, published in *Cellular and Molecular Neurobiology* (December 2003), reveal that p53 is failing to trigger apoptosis in those with autistic brain development. Further research has shown that insulin resistance is among the factors that dysregulate or block p53. If p53 malfunctions, tissues will be allowed to grow and exceed the DNA blueprint for a healthy brain. Increasingly, researchers are pursuing these leads aggressively, especially the clues to the common links among insulin resistance and autism, ADHD, schizophrenia, and bipolar disease.

In an article in *Medical Hypotheses* (2006, issue 2) lead author Kimberly A. Bazar of the San Mateo Medical Center in Palo Alto, California, wrote that "disparate conditions such as insulin resistance, diabetes, hypertension, syndrome X [metabolic syndrome], obesity, ADHD, depression, psychosis, sleep apnea, inflammation, autism, and schizophrenia may operate through common pathways, and treatments used exclusively for one of these conditions may prove beneficial for the others."

This is already proving to be true. Treatments for diabetes and metabolic syndrome are investigated to treat neurological disorders such as Alzheimer's disease and ADHD. But even if such medications provide such relief, the facts still point to the destructive effects of insulin resistance and metabolic syndrome, including on the brain. In fact, the growing understanding of how insulin resistance and metabolic syndrome affect the brain is giving new hope to children now suffering from ADHD.

COMBATING ADHD

Between 3 and 5 percent of all American children suffer from ADHD, and the incidence of the disorder is increasing. Since 1990, the sale of Ritalin and other drugs used to control the disorder have jumped fivefold. Increasingly, children are being placed on extremely powerful drugs that, in some cases, have significant side effects. Ritalin has been shown to cause liver cancer in laboratory animals, and some reports suggest that it may be associated with an increased risk of childhood depression.

For decades, parents of children with ADHD have noticed that their children's behavior improved dramatically when they avoided certain kinds of foods, including those that contain sugar, milk products, artificial colors, flavors, or preservatives. In the early 1970s, Benjamin Feingold, MD, an allergist who practiced in California, introduced the Feingold diet for children with ADHD. The diet restricted all foods that contained artificial colors, flavors, preservatives, and salicylates (aspirin-like substances that Dr. Feingold said could affect moods in sensitive children). Other foods and food substances were called into question as well, including milk products, corn, and wheat. Parents who adopted the Feingold diet said they saw immediate improvements in their children's behavior. In fact, communities and support groups sprang up throughout the country that swore by the effectiveness of Feingold's diet. Soon, scientific studies began investigating the approach.

To date, there have been twenty-three studies examining the relationship between specific food items and attention deficit and hyperactive behavior. "Some of these studies demonstrated significant improvement in the behavior of children when their diets were changed, or deterioration in their behavior when they were given food dyes or other offending foods," Eugene Arnold, professor emeritus of psychiatry at The Ohio State University told *Nutrition Action Healthletter*, a publication of Center for Science in the Public Interest (CSPI), a Washington, DC–based public advocacy group. "It makes a lot more sense to try modifying a child's diet before treating him or her with a stimulant drug," Dr. Marvin Boris, a New York pediatrician told CSPI some years earlier. Indeed, in a review of the research, CSPI found that fully seventeen of the twenty-three studies had reported a clear relationship between certain food substances and ADHD behaviors. Only six experiments had found no connection at all, CSPI reported.

Nevertheless, the food industry has seized upon the small doubt cast by those six studies to convince the general public that no relationship between food and behavior has been shown. Many medical experts today denounce the belief that food might play a role in either the onset or the severity of ADHD. They point to studies in which no relationship has been found between the two. Part of the problem has been that science could not explain how food components might affect brain function. Another issue is that researchers could not explain why some children might be sensitive to these substances, while others do not react to them.

All of that is now changing, especially as scientists are able to understand how food and exercise affect glucose, insulin, and brain function. Many researchers now believe that the relationship between food and ADHD may not be a straight line. Rather, there may be an interim set of conditions that must be established first in order for food to affect behavior, at least in a dramatic way as in the case of ADHD. That interim set of conditions may well start with insulin resistance and its partner in crime, inflammation.

"There is emerging evidence that insulin resistance triggers an inflammatory response in the central nervous system that, in turn, activates unique kinase pathways in neurons," said Jeffrey Bland, PhD, chief science officer for Metagenics, Inc., and Functional Medicine Research Center, both located in Gig Harbor, Washington. Dr. Bland is one of the world's leading experts on insulin and insulin signaling. "That means that anything that causes inflammation in the central nervous system, including excess sugar consumption, or sedentary lifestyle, or exposure to toxic heavy elements, can alter the inflammatory pathways, cause insulin resistance, and trigger kinase alterations," says Dr. Bland. Those changes in kinase patterns can, indeed, change the way the brain functions, which in turn can alter perception and behavior.

Several food substances lead to insulin resistance and inflammation, especially processed foods, sugar, and saturated fat—the very foods Dr. Feingold and others have identified as the causes of ADHD. Dr. Bland takes the theory even further. "All agents that the central nervous system perceives as 'foreign' might initiate an inflammatory response which in turn modifies kinase signaling, insulin sensitivity, and insulin signaling," he says.

Clearly, artificial colors, flavors, and preservatives are foreign to human biology, especially when you consider that they have only come into widespread use during the past forty years. The same might be said about the quantities of sugar and processed foods that we are eating today.

And although these substances are foreign to all of us, it's very possible that some children are genetically designed to be more sensitive to these substances than others. These sensitive children may be more vulnerable to insulin resistance and inflammation, which might make such conditions more acute, and thus result in more severe symptoms—including ADHD.

The relationship among food, lifestyle, and brain dysfunction is gaining increasing support from our growing understanding of signal transduction, which is revealing the underlying biology for how things go awry when insulin function is thrown off.

RACING TOWARD BURNOUT

The brain is a high-performance engine. Constantly monitoring every internal system and environmental event, the brain receives billions of bits of information during every instant, organizes the mass of data, and, in most cases, comes up with precisely the right response for the given condition or situation. It is a feat of computer engineering that may never be fully understood, much less matched by human invention.

All that activity, of course, requires energy—lots of it. In fact, your brain requires more glucose and oxygen than any other organ in your body—more than, say, your legs that carry you through each day, or your arms when you are lifting a heavy object. In order for the brain to utilize the available glucose, it must have insulin. But energy delivery is only one of insulin's important tasks. It also regulates how neurons function, which means it plays a key role in how you experience life.

Insulin increases a kinase enzyme known as Akt, which in turn decreases another enzyme, GSK-3. The seesaw of those two kinases—as one goes up, the other goes down—allows your brain to produce optimal amounts of the chemical neurotransmitter acetylcholine, which is essential for you to have memory and awareness of your surroundings—in short, cognition.

But acetylcholine is not the only crucial neurotransmitter regulated by insulin. Another is a substance called *glutamate*, which is responsible for creating states of arousal and excitement. Glutamate makes cells function more rapidly, much like pushing down on the gas pedal of your car and making the engine race. When glutamate is up, your brain functions much more rapidly.

All well and good, but if you've got too much glutamate, you're not going to be able to sit still for very long, or concentrate on anything for more than a few seconds. You've got to calm down in order to concentrate, to learn, to feel safe, and to enjoy the moment. Among its many duties, insulin regulates glutamate.

Unfortunately, when insulin isn't functioning properly in the brain, it creates complex problems that lead to brain dysfunction. Imagine cells that are forced to race all day and night, but at the same time are not given the raw materials they need to function properly. The engine races, but the materials needed for the cells to do their jobs—such as produce enough neurotransmitter for the brain to function properly—would be missing. Under such conditions, cells would race furiously for a time, burn out, and eventually die. You might experience a lot of arousal and then a big crash into depression. That's basically what happens when insulin cannot regulate glutamate properly. Here's how the problem plays out—at least as far as scientists understand it at this point.

THE BIOLOGY OF ANGUISH

Insulin controls glutamate by regulating an array of kinases. In health, insulin increases production of the kinase Akt, which in turn keeps GSK-3 from getting too high. If GSK-3 gets too high, your brain will produce more glutamate, which means more racing engine. In addition, insulin also promotes the production of a growth factor in the brain known as *brain-derived neurotrophic factor* (BDNF). BDNF actually buffers the toxic effects of glutamate— rather like eating a pastry in order to protect your stomach from the excess acids caused when you drink too much coffee. The effect of BDNF, therefore, is to protect your brain, in large part by protecting brain cells from the racing and burnout effects of glutamate.

In the insulin-resistant brain, there's plenty of glucose and insulin in the blood and tissue, but not enough of either enters the cells. As insulin and glucose drop off, BDNF drops. Akt levels also drop, which means GSK-3 goes up. That, in turn, drives ups glutamate. Now cells are racing.

Interestingly, BDNF levels are significantly lower in depressed patients and in those with other psychiatric conditions. And antidepressants are effective based on their ability to raise BDNF. Furthermore, BDNF has been demonstrated to have antidiabetic effects because the protein enhances insulin sensitivity.

All of which means that BDNF protects your brain cells, slows things down against racing and burnout, and thereby protects against depression and other mental disorders. But this crucial protein depends on proper insulin functioning. Researchers have found that when glucose and insulin metabolism is impaired, BDNF levels drop. That means that one of the brain's primary protectors has been diminished and is in low supply, thus making the brain susceptible to numerous types of mental disorders. The relationship between insulin and BDNF may well be the crucial link between insulin resistance and psychiatric conditions.

Scientists speculate that for people with bipolar disease, the rising tide of glutamate causes the brain to be aroused, agitated, and on high alert. The mind is racing, the body nervous and wanting to move. For the adult with bipolar disorder, elevated glutamate is one of the fuels for the mania—that high that inevitably crashes into depression. For the autistic child, the rising glutamate brings on symptoms of hyperactivity along with anxiety, loss of control, and withdrawal.

Whenever there is racing of cells—the consequence of too much glutamate—there are going to be exhaust fumes. In the brain's case, that means lots of oxidation, free radicals, and inflammation. Immune cells arrive in the brain tissue and attempt to clear the free radicals, but whenever immune cells show up in large numbers, they themselves produce inflammatory cytokines, oxidants, and free radicals, all of which can heighten the levels of inflammation, including in the brain.

Dr. Bland points out that that inflammation even further throws off GSK-3, which means that you're going to get even higher glutamate levels, greater metabolic activity, heightened arousal, and all of the inflammation-related side effects.

Keep in mind that both ends of the age spectrum are affected by these imbalances. For the young person, there is much greater risk of ADHD and, for those who are genetically vulnerable, greater possibility of schizophrenia or bipolar disorder. For the elderly person, the elevated inflammation and higher GSK-3 means lower acetylcholine, poorer memory, and greater risk of Alzheimer's disease.

Currently, there are several drugs used being investigated to treat ADHD, Alzheimer's, bipolar disorder, and autism, which are designed to reign in GSK-3. Lithium is a good example. Lithium not only dampens glutamate, but it also protects the cell from destroying itself as a consequence of glutamate-induced racing. That, in turn, will lower glutamate levels. Various compounds are able to modulate the toxic effects of glutamate, and are either currently in use or under investigation for the treatment of a diverse set of clinical conditions, including Alzheimer's disease (memantine), migraines (topirimate and valproic acid), bipolar disease (valproic acid, lamotrigine), epilepsy (topirimate, valproic acid, lamotrigine), and chronic pain (gabapentin and pregabalin).

As needed as these drugs are, none of them gets to the real source of the problem. In effect, they deal with the wrong end of the disorder. The real source of the problem may be insulin resistance, which sets the dominoes in motion. The fact that individual drugs work on the same kinase and neurotransmitters and are effective in the treatment of multiple disorders has led many researchers to believe that these disorders spring from the same root system.

NEUROTRANSMITTERS

In the human body, nothing happens independently. Everything is dependent, it seems, on everything else. The human mind cannot fathom the awesome orchestration of trillions of cells, each performing multiple tasks, and all of it woven together into a moving tapestry that is both orderly and creative at the same time. As you've no doubt noticed, that tapestry gets scrambled by metabolic syndrome.

Among the relationships that scientists have recognized consistently is that people with metabolic syndrome suffer from heart disease as well as depression. As researchers looked more closely for clues as to why insulin resistance might be associated with depression, they found an interesting fact turn up again and again. People with metabolic syndrome have low serotonin levels.

Serotonin is responsible for creating within us a sense of well-being and confidence. When elevated, serotonin gives us the ability to concentrate, to focus on a given subject, and to relax and enjoy deep sleep. When serotonin is low, we can experience increased anxiety and, if it falls low enough, even depression.

Most of the antidepressant drugs are referred to as "selective serotonin re-uptake inhibitors (SSRI)." These drugs work by increasing brain levels of serotonin, and thereby lower depression.

Serotonin can also be elevated by eating carbohydrates. Carbohydrates increase blood levels of an amino acid called tryptophan, which in turn elevates serotonin in the brain. Usually, brain levels of serotonin are increased within twenty minutes of eating a high-carbohydrate meal, such as a whole grain, or bread, or a dessert that contains carbohydrates. Foods that contain rapidly absorbed carbohydrates, such as sugar and processed foods, provide a rapid elevation of serotonin. But because these sugars are burned off or stored very quickly, both the blood sugar and the serotonin levels fall off just as quickly. We get a quick high, but we are soon feeling low and depleted. As serotonin levels fall, we can feel more anxious and even a bit depressed.

Foods that contain slowly absorbed carbohydrates from unprocessed foods such as whole-grain brown rice, barley, and millet, and from pulpy vegetables such as squash and sweet potatoes, provide more long-lasting energy and long-lasting serotonin levels.

It's worth remembering, as well, that slowly absorbed carbohydrates do not create that glucose and insulin spike that is associated with weight gain and eventually insulin resistance. That's why these foods are frequently recommended to treat weight, insulin resistance, metabolic syndrome, and diabetes.

Serotonin's opposite is dopamine, which, like glutamate, creates states of heightened arousal and alertness. Dopamine is essential for mental focus and rapid movement. It gives us a greater sense of concentration and energy. When dopamine levels become elevated, we can experience heightened alertness, increased aggression, increased energy, and an inability to sit still. As dopamine continues to increase, a person can feel increased anxiety and fear. At even higher elevations, paranoia is common.

Dopamine is rapidly elevated when we eat a meal made up of high-protein foods such as beef, pork, eggs, and fish. These foods boost blood levels of an amino acid called *tyrosine*, which in turn raises brain levels of dopamine. Usually, dopamine rises quite significantly within twenty minutes of eating a high-protein meal.

Scientists have known for many years that insulin resistance and coronary heart disease were both associated with depression, though the reasons for this connection have remained a mystery. Further research revealed that people with insulin resistance and metabolic syndrome have much lower levels of serotonin in their brains, which explains, at least in part, why they would be depressed. Though the exact signaling has yet to be worked out, it's possible that insulin resistance could block neurons from producing enough serotonin.

Insulin resistance prevents adequate glucose—the source of which is carbohydrates—from getting to cells. In this way, insulin resistance could disrupt the conversion of carbohydrates into tryptophan, which in turn could prevent the brain from producing adequate serotonin. This, of course, would result in a decline in feelings of well-being. If serotonin falls low enough, depression will set in. This theory is supported by recent data that demonstrated a significantly higher rate of depression in overweight individuals.

Insulin is involved in every single function of human biology. It is the gatekeeper to our cells. Disturb insulin function and you disrupt the workings of our cells, no matter where they are located—in the liver, or pancreas, or heart, or coronary arteries, or the brain. Insulin is either the basis for our health or our Achilles' heel. There is no escaping its influence, or its power to determine our fate.

While scientists search for answers to ADHD, schizophrenia, bipolar disorder, and even autism, we possess a power to help ourselves heal. That power lies in controlling our insulin levels through our daily behavior. One of the best ways to do that, and at the same time promote optimal mood and brain function, is to adopt a Mediterranean diet. Researchers are consistently finding that the omega-3 fatty acids in fish oils, flax seed oils, walnuts, canola oil, and olive oil optimize insulin function and have an antidepressant effect.

The Mediterranean diet is rich in fish and seafood—excellent sources of omega-3 fatty acids—and low in processed foods, thus offering lower levels of omega-6 fats and specifically arachidonic acid. Also, Mediterranean people use olive oil to cook, as opposed to safflower, corn, and sunflower oils, all rich in omega-6s and specifically arachidonic acid. Researchers have consistently found that people who follow a more Mediterranean-like diet have more stable and brighter moods than those who eat a diet rich in processed foods and oils rich in omega-6s. The dietary program described in chapters 11 and 12 can raise your omega-3 levels and lower your omega-6s, thus elevating your insulin sensitivity, elevating your mood, and enhancing your brain function.

· 10 ·

Assessing Your Insulin Levels

The behaviors that affect our insulin levels are so familiar to many of us that we take them for granted. The common side effects of high glucose and high insulin—weight gain, along with fluctuations in energy and mood—are often viewed as the normal effects of aging, or a temporary phase that we may be going through. All too often, the small warning signs are neglected. Gradually, the conditions get worse until the day when we realize that something is very wrong and we're suddenly thrown into crisis.

Following is a simple checklist, along with some of the medical signs and symptoms, that can alert you to the possibility that your glucose and insulin levels may be too high and that it's time to change your behaviors. The first part of this checklist is a series of questions that will give you a good, clear picture of the ordinary symptoms that high insulin—and especially insulin resistance—can cause. The questions can serve as an important tool for reflecting on your overall health and providing the basis for an informative discussion you can have with your doctor.

Following the list of questions is information on a series of blood tests that your doctor can administer to determine if you are, indeed, insulin resistant. Once your doctor knows the specifics of your condition, he or she can offer medications and a diet and lifestyle that can bring your insulin back into normal ranges, and in the process restore your health.

Both the questions and the suggested medical tests are provided by Mark Hyman, MD, who is currently the editor-in-chief of *Alternative Therapies in Health and Medicine*, a peer-reviewed medical journal that covers mainstream and alternative approaches to medicine and health care. Dr. Hyman is the former co–medical director of Canyon Ranch, an acclaimed health resort in the Berkshires. He is also a *New York Times* bestselling author; his many books include *The UltraSimple Diet: Kick-Start Your Metabolism and Safely Lose Up to 10 Pound in 7 Days* and *Ultraprevention: The 6-Week Plan That Will Make You Healthy for Life.*

• • •

Let's begin with the questions. Give yourself one point for each positive answer. If your score totals five or higher, you should consult your physician and, under his or her guidance, make immediate changes in your diet and exercise habits.

Blood Sugar Problems (Insulin resistance)

1. I crave sweets, eat them, and though I get a temporary boost of energy and mood, I later crash.
2. I have a family history of diabetes, hypoglycemia, or alcoholism.
3. I get irritable, anxious, tired, and jittery or get headaches intermittently throughout the day, but feel better temporarily after meals.
4. I get dizzy when I stand up quickly.
5. I feel shaky two to three hours after a meal.
6. I eat a low-fat diet and can't seem to lose weight.
7. If I miss a meal I feel cranky and irritable, weak, or tired.
8. If I eat a carbohydrate breakfast (muffin, bagel, cereal, pancakes, etc.), I can't seem to control my eating for the rest of the day.
9. Once I start eating sweets or carbohydrates, I can't seem to stop.
10. If I eat fish or meat and vegetables I feel good, but I seem to get sleepy or feel "drugged" after eating a meal full of pasta, bread, potatoes, and dessert.
11. I go for the bread basket at the restaurant.
12. I get heart palpitations after eating sweets.
13. I seem salt sensitive (I tend to retain water).
14. I get panic attacks in the afternoon if I skip breakfast.
15. Without my morning coffee, I can't get going in the morning.
16. I am often moody, impatient, or anxious.
17. My memory and concentration are poor.

18. Eating makes me calm.

19. I get tired a few hours after eating.

20. I get night sweats.

21. I am frequently thirsty.

22. I seem to get frequent infections.

23. I am tired most of the time.

24. I have extra weight around the middle.

25. My hair is thin in the places I don't want it to be thin and grows in the places it shouldn't.

26. I have chronic fungal infections (jock itch, vaginal yeast infections, dry scaly patches on my skin).

I have these diseases, as diagnosed by a medical professional:

27. Polycystic ovarian syndrome or infertility

28. High blood pressure

29. Heart disease

30. Diabetes (adult onset)

31. Dementia

32. Cancer

My blood tests are:

33. Low HDL levels (<50 for men, <60 for women)

34. High triglycerides (>100)

35. Triglyceride/HDL ratio of greater than 5

36. Abnormal liver function tests or fatty liver

37. High serum ferritin (>200)

38. High serum uric acid (>7.0)

39. Low serum magnesium (<2.0)

40. Fasting blood sugar (>90)

41. Fasting insulin (>8)
42. (Poor glucose/insulin tolerance test result)

My sugar intake is:

43. Excessive—I crave and have sweets daily, and drink more than two sweetened or artificially sweetened drinks a day and eat foods with high fructose corn syrup (food bars, processed food, etc.).
44. High—I eat my share of sugar and sweet foods, crave them, and feel like it is a constant struggle to cut down.
45. Moderate—I treat myself occasionally to sweets (zero to three times a week).
46. Low—I don't crave or want sugars and eat them very infrequently.

In choosing carbohydrates in my diet, I generally pick:

47. Whole grains such as brown rice, quinoa, whole wheat, 100 percent rye, sweet potatoes, squashes, or whole-grain breads or pastas.
48. White food such as white bread, white rice, bagels, pasta, white potatoes, popcorn, common breakfast cereals.

If you answered "no" to question 47, add a point to your total score; if you answered "yes" to question 47, do not add a point.

If you answered "yes" to question 48, add a point to your total score; if you answered "no" to question 48, do not add a point to your score.

BASIC TESTING FOR
BLOOD SUGAR IMBALANCE

If, after taking the test, you feel that it would be wise to see your physician, the following tests are among those he or she will want to do to determine if your glucose and insulin levels are excessive, and if you are insulin resistant.

Blood Cholesterol and Triglycerides, also known as a Lipid Profile

Your total blood cholesterol should be less than 180 milligrams per deciliter of blood (written as 180 mg/dl).

Your high-density lipoprotein (the good cholesterol) should be greater than 60 mg/dl.

Your triglycerides should be less than 100 mg/dl.

Fasting Glucose and Insulin Tests, accompanied by 1-hour and 2-hour Post-Fasting Tests

Your fasting glucose should be less than 90.

Your fasting insulin level should be less than 5.

Your 1-hour and 2-hour insulin level should be less than 25.

Your 1-hour and 2-hour glucose should be less than 120.

Hemoglobin

Hemoglobin is the primary component of red blood cells, and carries oxygen within the blood. Doctors run tests on specific fractions of the hemoglobin. Have your doctor test your A1C (HbA1c). It should be less than 5.5.

Fibrinogen

Fibrinogen is a clotting protein produced by the liver. If it becomes excessively elevated, it can lead to increased clots and an increased risk of heart attack and stroke. People with insulin resistance often have higher than normal fibrinogen, one of the many reasons they are at an increased risk of heart attack and stroke. Your fibrinogen level should be lower than 300 mg/dl.

Uric Acid

Your kidneys filter uric acid from the blood. People who eat diets rich in animal proteins and fats tend to have high uric acid levels, which can damage the kidneys and lead to gout. Your uric acid level should be lower than 5.0.

High-sensitivity C-reactive Protein

C-reactive protein is a test that can determine the general level of inflammation throughout your body. It can predict your risk of heart disease and other serious illnesses. Your high-sensitivity C-reactive protein level should be less than 0.7.

Ferritin

Ferritin is a protein in the body that stores iron. High iron levels are associated with an array of illnesses, including cancer. Your ferritin level should be less than 200 milligrams per milliliter of blood.

Liver Function Tests

High glucose, high insulin, and metabolic syndrome are all associated with decreased liver function. Your doctor will want to run a series of liver function tests on you, including those known by ALT, AST, and GGT. All three should be within normal limits.

Homocysteine

Homocysteine is an amino acid that rises when we consume excess levels of animal protein. It combines with LDL cholesterol to form a highly inflammatory compound that increases the risk of heart disease. Your homocysteine levels should be less than 8 mg/dl.

Testosterone Levels in Men

Male testosterone levels should be greater than 500 mg/dl.

Free-floating testosterone should be greater than 60 mg/dl.

DHEA-Sulfate Levels in Women

DHEA-sulfate (Dehydroepiandrosterone-sulfate) is an important steroid hormone produced in the body. It is further converted to testosterone in men and estrogen in women. Women with elevated levels of DHEA-sulfate often suffer from adrenal exhaustion and polycystic ovaries. DHEA-sulfate should be within normal limits (ranges vary depending on the laboratory).

• • •

The questions and tests provided here can tell you if you are at risk of having high insulin and even insulin resistance. Only your doctor can confirm your suspicions. That's why we recommend that if you have any of the symptoms described in the questionnaire, you should see your physician as soon as possible. We also recommend that you adopt the diet and lifestyle described in the next chapters.

· 11 ·

Controlling Your Insulin Levels

We should all be asking ourselves what can we do to protect ourselves and our loved ones from the multiple epidemics that arise from insulin resistance.

We started this book by explaining the delicate process upon which human health rests—signal transduction, the passing of information within and between cells. And that understanding, it turns out, is both the alpha and the omega of our dilemma today. The illnesses we suffer from today are caused by bad information being passed to cells, which in turn alters the function of our genes, with terrible consequences. Our solution lies in changing the information that our cells and genes receive. We can do that by changing the types of food we eat and by exercising daily.

For the past fifty years, nutrition science has been dominated by the language of fats, carbohydrates, calories, vitamins, minerals, and fiber. Today, a new understanding of food and its effects on our bodies is emerging. That new science sees food, literally, as packages of information. The food items that we recognize as beef, whole grains, pasta, or vegetables are, from the standpoint of our cells, bunches of code, packages of information. The nutrients and phytochemicals in food serve as commands at the cellular and genetic levels. Those commands regulate gene expression and thus every bodily function.

Scientists are now finding that foods created largely in factories present our bodies with very different types of information than those produced by nature. From the standpoint of our cells, that Krispy Kreme doughnut presents a very different set of command codes than, say, a couple of slices of whole-grain bread.

Things get far more complicated, and thus far more dangerous, when bits of information are introduced into our bodies that are extremely foreign to our biology. We're talking about all those artificial flavors, colors, preservatives, and pesticides that are prevalent throughout our food. These, too, are tiny packets of information that affect the way our cells and genes function. The problem is that they are giving the wrong messages, signals, and instruction.

"Our food contains all kinds of additives, emulsifiers, and preservatives, and these substances send information to the body that our genes are not used to receiving," says Dr. Jeff Bland, one of the nation's leading scientists specializing in the study of how food affects human genes.

"The genes that are turned on as a consequence of the foods that we eat today are the genes that might be collectively and symbolically known as those of Mars, the god of war," says Dr. Bland. "The color is red, which is a symbol for inflammation. The signal is alarm. The foods we eat are causing widespread alarm throughout the system." And that alarm is triggering chemical changes throughout the body that lead to disease and premature death.

The primary source of that alarm, of course, is processed foods—foods that have been altered from their original state and have had their calories packed and concentrated into smaller and smaller packages. Processed foods, with their calories and their chemicals, have the body seeing red.

WHY HEALTH IS DECLINING SO RAPIDLY

For most of human experience, we consumed food essentially in its natural state—in the case of plant foods, directly from the branch, vine, stem, and root; in the case of animal foods, directly from the bones of the animals we killed. These were, indeed, the first "natural foods"—no artificial anything.

Cooking, of course, was the first form of food processing, but even that did not occur during the first 1.5 million years of our evolution. In fact, no one knows for certain when our earliest ancestors started cooking food, but we probably got the idea when game was roasted in a forest fire and one of our curious forebears put the blackened carcass in his mouth. The first of our cave-dwelling relatives to use fire to prepare food was probably *Homo erectus*, who lived some 700,000 years ago, but scientists debate when he might have started barbecuing. It could have come as late as 400,000 years ago.

From there, it took a very long time for the art of food processing to arise. The Egyptians began making bread and beer around 5000

BCE, some 7,000 years ago. The people of mid- and lower Asia—today's Iraq, Iran, and Afghanistan—began making cheese around the same time. About 4,500 years later, at around 2500 BCE, the Chinese began to process and produce salt, an art that was further refined in India a thousand years later. Sugar, derived from sugar cane, didn't appear until 500 BCE, again in India.

Every culture has had its own form of food processing. The Chinese, Japanese, and Indonesians brought food processing to a high art with the development of bean products such as miso, shoyu, tamari, tempeh, and tofu, just to name a handful. Many more foods the world over were derived from whole grains. For the most part, food processing, no matter how creative, was minimal, meaning that the food itself was not significantly altered from its original state. The grain for bread was crushed and sifted a bit, but the bread itself retained much of its fiber and nutrient content; there were no artificial preservatives introduced to improve shelf life, no colors to enhance appearance. The foods were not fortified with synthetically derived nutrients, nor did they lose many nutrients during processing. There were no artificial emulsifiers, nor artificial forms of fat such as hydrogenated oils and trans fats, which are common in processed foods today.

In a very real sense, the information conveyed in traditionally processed foods was essentially the same as that derived from nature's food. Traditional processing maintained the essential integrity of the food, and therefore the integrity of the information flowing to the body.

That all began to change in the United States in the 1950s.

There are many forms of processing that are carried out today.

But for the most part, processing means taking a large quantity of food, cooking it, removing the fiber and many nutrients, drying it, and concentrating the calories into a smaller volume of food. For example, corn, a relatively low-calorie food, is transformed into corn chips, a high-calorie food. Wheat, another low-calorie food, is used to make rolls and bagels, both much richer in calories. Very often, food manufacturers add fat to processed foods, which drives up the calorie content even further. Potato chips, cookies, pastries, and muffins are common examples.

In most cases, processing also means introducing synthetically created chemicals in the form of preservatives that will allow a food to keep from decaying—going bad—while on your grocery shelf. In addition, many different flavors, colors, and fats are added to enhance taste and appearance.

One of the lessons we are learning from our experience with processed foods is that the more artificial the food, the more foreign—and therefore more harmful—the information flowing to the body. Trans fats are a good example. A study published in the September 2002 issue of *The Journal of Nutrition* reported that trans fats significantly increase insulin resistance, inflammation, overweight, and the risk of both diabetes and heart disease. Researchers at the Harvard School of Public Health have found that each 2 percent increase in trans fats raises a woman's risk of coronary disease by 93 percent. By comparison, the researchers have found that for every 5 percent increase in saturated fat, a woman's chances of having heart disease increases 17 percent.

Then there is the addition of sugar and artificial flavors, all of which are designed to arouse taste buds. In many cases, caffeine and other substances have been added to heighten that arousal even further.

WAY TOO MUCH INFORMATION FOR THE BODY TO HANDLE

In a very real sense, processed foods assault the body with far too much information. The overabundance of calories, saturated fat, and artificial ingredients is essentially a media blitz on our cells. That avalanche of information has widespread effects on our biology. Shortly after consuming a meal containing processed foods, we find the blood engorged with too much glucose, too much cholesterol, too many triglycerides, and too much inflammation. All of these factors disrupt insulin signaling throughout the body, including the nervous system and brain.

Excess information is confusing to both our senses and our cells. Walk into Times Square after dark and you will find yourself overwhelmed with lights, colors, noise, heights, faces, and bodies in motion. In time, you may become inured to the explosion of information flowing to your senses, but it's unlikely that you will ever be able to fully comprehend it, or make order out of it.

The modern diet is having a similar effect on our bodies. Like drugs, our food today is manufactured to create peak experiences. The body is instantly ablaze with inflammatory compounds and excitatory hormones and neurotransmitters, all of which change mood and alter our perceptions.

As with all drugs, rapid elevations are followed by precipitous falls. Blood sugar and neurochemistry levels drop, causing declines in energy, mood, and mental function. A wide array of physical and mental disorders is among the consequences of this roller-coaster ride in blood sugar, hormones, and neurotransmitters. Once these lows set in, the brain triggers cravings for the addictive food substances—whether it's a hamburger, or a milk shake, or a sugary snack.

Nowhere have the addictive and destructive effects of our modern diet been better demonstrated—at least anecdotally—than by Morgan Spurlock's 2004 documentary film, *Super Size Me.* Spurlock, who at the time was thirty-three years old, went on a thirty-day diet that consisted entirely of food sold at McDonald's. Before going on the diet, he underwent extensive medical examination by three medical doctors, all of whom proclaimed him in excellent health. Those same physicians followed Spurlock closely during his month-long ordeal and documented his steady—not to mention terrifying—decline in health. Blood tests revealed a precipitous rise in cholesterol, triglycerides, and inflammation, as well as an equally dramatic decline in liver function. After Spurlock was on the McDonald's diet for a couple of weeks, one of his doctors told him that his liver functions resembled that of an alcoholic's. If he continued, his doctor warned him, his liver would fail. Meanwhile, Spurlock rapidly gained weight, suggesting that he was becoming increasingly insulin resistant.

In addition to the measurable declines in health, Spurlock also experienced depression and a decline in energy and mental and sexual function.

Remarkably, even as his health was failing, Spurlock admitted that he found himself craving the McDonald's food, and that he needed more and more of it to cause the same kinds of emotional highs and feelings of well-being that were associated with the food. He was becoming addicted to McDonald's fast-food blend of fatty meats, soft buns, sugary soft drinks, and desserts.

Children throughout the United States find themselves in this same dilemma: They're addicted to foods that are causing them to be overweight, insulin resistant, and prediabetic—if not fully diabetic already.

"The conditions we have today—that is, a diet and lifestyle that create insulin resistance and inflammation—are the reasons why we are seeing an increase in dementia, brain inflammation, non-alcoholic inflammatory hepatitis, cardiovascular disease, and many common cancers," says Dr. Bland. "All of these are manifestations of the information molecules that come from a diet that was really manufactured for the purpose of shelf stability, and not for the purpose of nutrition and health."

Therein lies the problem. The economics of convenience, of shelf life, of instant gratification—these are the driving forces that are actually creating our food supply today. Our multiple epidemics testify to their effects.

For two million years, nature determined our food choices. Today, economic forces and food manufacturers determine to a great extent what we eat. With that change have come new, foreign commands to our cells and genes, with chaotic and deadly effects.

"As the population ages, we're going to see even greater numbers of people suffering from these very diseases, which, many economists predict, will have catastrophic effects on our health care system," says Dr. Bland.

INFORMATION OVERLOAD

Just as processed foods overwhelm us with certain kinds of data, they also convey too little of the kinds of information the body has grown accustomed to receiving, and depends upon for health. Scientists have yet to identify and understand all the chemicals in any given plant food. A single stalk of broccoli, for example, is said to contain literally thousands of phytochemicals. It's possible that every one of those substances plays an important role in human health. In fact, according to Dr. Bland, unprocessed animal and plant foods contain substances that actually regulate every one of our genes and biological functions.

"When you think about the kinds of foods—and hence the kinds of information—on which we evolved, you must consider that the diet was composed of unprocessed proteins and plants, and that such a diet was consumed over many, many millennia," says Dr. Bland. "Over time, a symbiosis developed between our food and the workings of our genes.

"Plant foods are enormously complex. They contain a rich array of minerals, flavonoids, polyphenols, nucleic acids, tecopherols, and tens of thousands of other phytochemicals. As we ate these foods and evolved, we came to depend on these substances in order to regulate gene expression and sustain health. Rather than create messages from the god of war, these foods send very different messages to our genes. They create signaling processes that regulate insulin sensitivity. They regulate cell division and repair. They determine GI function—our ability to absorb nutrients and eliminate waste. They determine the strength and balance of the immune system, and consequently regulate inflammatory responses. All of these functions are harmoniously controlled by eating a diet that is composed of foods that we refer to as minimally processed."

All of these chemicals—which number in the tens of thousands—cannot be provided by a supplement, or any form of food fortification. The only way these compounds can be obtained is by consuming a wide variety of plant foods and unprocessed animal proteins. Like many other health experts, Dr. Bland points to the Mediterranean diet as an ideal model. "In the Mediterranean diet, animal protein is not the centerpiece, as it is in the American diet," says Dr. Bland. "Vegetables, beans, and whole-grain products are the center of the diet. And everything is minimally processed. And if you look at the health of people who follow such a diet, you see that they have lower rates of the common illnesses than we do on a highly processed, meat-centered diet."

Traditional diets around the world have many similarities in common. The Asian diet, like the Mediterranean, is centered around plant foods and supplemented by animal proteins. So, too, were many African and South American diets. The foods throughout the traditional world are minimally processed and nutritionally rich. And not surprisingly, the populations who live on them experience low rates of the illnesses that are skyrocketing in the United States and other modern countries.

Such traditional diets are delicious, satisfying, and easy to adopt. Indeed, they are also the foundation of our health.

SUPPLEMENTS

It's important to remember that the first and second steps to the full recovery of our health are a healthy diet and an exercise program. Nothing can replace those two steps if we are really committed to overcoming the illnesses we now face. However, we can also get some help from certain nutrients that, when administered correctly, can increase insulin sensitivity, reduce inflammation, and help fight major illnesses. Some may also improve the overall quality of life.

Since many people who are already ill may want to experiment with these nutrients, we urge you to consult your physician before taking any supplement, whether it is described here or anywhere else. Only your doctor can tell you if these substances will interact safely with any medications you may be taking, or if the doses you may be contemplating are safe for your condition.

Research has consistently shown that, when taken in the right doses, and under the right conditions, the three forms of supplementation described below may well prove beneficial to people suffering from insulin resistance and its related disorders.

Vitamin D

Known as the "sunshine vitamin," vitamin D is actually a hormone produced by the body when exposed to sunlight. Vitamin D is available in certain foods such as sardines and fortified milk products. Though traditionally seen as essential for strong bones and teeth, vitamin D has been increasingly recognized as important in a whole range of illnesses. Researchers have long noted that cancer rates are lowest in parts of the world with the highest exposure to sunlight—areas such as the southern United States, and all regions closer to the equator.

Recently, scientists have found that vitamin D deficiency is also associated with higher rates of insulin resistance, diabetes, heart diseases, high blood pressure, parathyroid dysfunction, and end-stage renal disease. When people with low vitamin D levels receive supplements of the nutrient, their glucose metabolism and insulin sensitivity are improved. For many, blood pressure is also lowered.

Most people require about fifteen minutes of sunlight on their face, hands, and arms to obtain adequate amounts of vitamin D. However, as we age, our ability to produce vitamin D declines, so people over the age of sixty may require supplementation of vitamin D in order to get adequate amounts.

Vitamin D is fat soluble and therefore is stored in the body over time. By the time a person reaches seventy years of age, his or her vitamin D production falls to about 30 percent of what it was when he or she was twenty-five. That also means that many seniors will require some supplementation. The recommended dietary allowance (RDA) for people younger than fifty is 200 International Units (IU) per day, but researchers recommend that people between fifty and seventy get 400 IU daily, and those over seventy get as much as 600 IU each day.

Calcium and Vitamin D

A study done by researchers at Harvard University's Brigham and Women's Hospital in Boston (published in *Diabetes Care*, December 2005) examined the effects of calcium and vitamin D levels in more than 10,000 women. The researchers found that those women with the highest intakes of calcium and vitamin D had the lowest rates of metabolic syndrome. Interestingly, the scientists found that only when vitamin D was taken with calcium was it associated with lower rates of metabolic syndrome.

Calcium is easily obtained from many sources, including green and leafy vegetables (collard greens provide 300 mg per cup), sardines (3 ounces provide 325 mg), soy milk (300 mg per cup), skim milk and skim milk products (300 mg per cup), fortified orange juice (350 mg per cup), tofu ($1/4$ block provides 145 mg), cooked soybeans (260 mg per cup), and almonds (70 mg in 1 ounce). The RDA for people under fifty is 1,000 milligrams (mg) per day; for people older than fifty, the RDA is 1,200 mg.

Most nutrition experts recommend that if you supplement, you do not go above 500 mg per day, largely because the body has trouble assimilating doses higher than that level. Calcium supplementation of 2,000 mg or higher may cause kidney stones and other kidney related problems.

Alpha-Lipoic Acid

An antioxidant found in many plant and animal foods, alpha-lipoic acid (ALA) is used by the body to produce energy. It supports and protects mitochondrial function. It also protects DNA from damage from free radicals.

Scientists only recently began studying the antioxidant, but the results so far have been very exciting. It has been shown to improve insulin sensitivity and reduce body weight, and may be effective in the treatment of diabetes, heart disease, stroke, and Alzheimer's and Parkinson's diseases. Some studies have shown that it improves muscle strength, energy levels, brain function, and immune response. A study published in the medical journal *Biochemical and Biophysical Research Communications* (July 8, 2005) showed that supplementation of ALA reduced body weight and lowered triglycerides in the muscles of laboratory animals. The researchers also showed that it prevented diabetes in diabetes-prone obese rats. Other research has shown that ALA is highly anti-inflammatory.

Doctors in Germany are already prescribing ALA in the treatment of type 2 diabetes, heart disease, stroke, multiple sclerosis, HIV, nerve damage, and Parkinson's and Alzheimer's diseases.

Researchers have most often used doses between 100 and 600 mg per day, but higher doses have also been used to beneficial effect. Increasingly, U.S. scientists and informed medical doctors are recommending it be taken with diabetes medication. Consult your physician before taking ALA, but for those with insulin-resistant illnesses, the antioxidant is worth investigating.

GENERAL DIETARY RECOMMENDATIONS TO RESTORE INSULIN SENSITIVITY AND LOWER INFLAMMATION

Researchers are now virtually unanimous in their recommendation that we adopt a diet that is based largely on plant foods. The reasons are many, but here are some of the most important.

1. They are lower in calories.

Plant foods, rich in fiber and water, will fill you up and keep your calorie intake down. They will cause you to lose weight, if you are overweight, or keep your weight low, without causing hunger.

- Unprocessed whole grains such as brown rice, barley, millet, oats, and quinoa. A three and a half ounce serving of boiled brown rice contains approximately 130 calories. Oatmeal, barley, millet, and quinoa are even lower in calorie content. Eat at least two servings per day of whole, unprocessed grains. Serving size doesn't matter. Simply eat until you are satisfied. A diet dominated by whole foods—whole grains, vegetables, and fruit—will allow you to be fully sated and at the same time will promote optimal, healthy weight.

- Green and leafy vegetables such as bok choy, broccoli, Brussels sprouts, collard greens, kale, mustard greens, watercress. (A full list is provded in the next chapter.) Vegetables, as we have already seen, are extremely low in calories. A pound of broccoli, 130 calories; a pound of lentil beans, 530; a pound of cauliflower, 110; a pound of spinach, 100. Eat at least three servings of green and leafy vegetables daily. Serving size doesn't matter. Eat until you are satisfied.

- Squash, tubers, and roots. Like green and leafy vegetables, they are low in calories and rich in nutrition. Eat at least one serving per day of sweet vegetables, such as squash, tubers, or roots.

- Beans. Four servings per week.

- Fruit. At least one serving per day.

Contrast these numbers with high-fat animal foods (fried chicken with the skin, 1,190 calories per pound; hot dogs, 1,500 calories per pound) and processed foods (Stouffer's French

Bread Pizza, 1,098 calories, or Health Valley fat-free whole-wheat crackers, 1,620 calories).

As we have already seen, weight loss changes the types of hormones produced by the adipose tissue, especially adiponectin, a substance that protects us against insulin resistance, cardiovascular disease, and various forms of cancer.

2. They are slowly absorbed, keeping insulin levels low.

Whole, unprocessed grains, beans, vegetables, and fruit contain long chains of complex carbohydrates that are encased in long strands of fiber. In order for the carbohydrates to be released from the fibrous matrix, they must be worked on by the intestine, a process that takes hours. Gradually, these sugars are dripped into the bloodstream, causing a steady flow of energy to the body. All of which means that these foods are slowly absorbed. They keep glucose and insulin levels low to normal. They lower inflammation and promote insulin sensitivity, weight loss, and cardiovascular health.

The simple sugars found in processed foods, on the other hand, are rapidly absorbed into the bloodstream. Some of the sugars in a candy bar, for example, are absorbed into the bloodstream through the tongue. Once in the blood, these simple sugars cause a rapid rise in glucose and insulin levels, which in turn lead to high levels of blood fats, weight gain, and eventually to insulin resistance.

3. They are low in saturated fat and trans fats, which makes them anti-inflammatory.

Saturated and trans fats are two of the most inflammatory substances in the food supply, and thus are part of the reason we suffer from the pandemic in degenerative diseases. Most unprocessed plant foods are extremely low in saturated fat. Moreover, they contain no trans fats (only processed foods contain these types of fats).

4. Plant foods contain fats that promote weight loss.

As we saw in chapter 4, plant foods, rich in polyunsaturated and monounsaturated fats, increase production of the hormone leptin, which enhances insulin sensitivity and promotes weight loss.

5. They are rich in phytochemicals that reduce inflammation and prevent disease.

Plant foods are the most abundant sources of substances that boost the immune system, protect cells from insult and mutation, lower cholesterol, and improve circulation to cells throughout the body.

A comprehensive list of anti-inflammatory foods is provided below. In addition, you will want to adopt an exercise program that will help you lose weight and fight inflammation and insulin resistance.

EXERCISE FOR MAXIMUM INSULIN SENSITIVITY, WEIGHT LOSS, AND PROTECTION FROM DISEASE

Exercise is highly anti-inflammatory. It also dramatically improves insulin sensitivity. You do not have to strain yourself in order to gain the benefits of exercise. A daily thirty-minute walk will lower insulin, burn fat, and lower inflammation. If you cannot walk for thirty minutes, three ten-minute walks will have the same cumulative effects as a thirty-minute stroll.

The best exercise program, however, is composed of three parts.

1. A daily walk of thirty minutes or more.
2. Engage in a physical activity that you enjoy two or three times per week. This could be a sport such as tennis, basketball, racketball, swimming, canoeing, or kayaking. It could be a martial art, such as Tai Chi Chuan, chi gong, karate, or aikido. Take a yoga class or a course in ballroom dancing, tango, swing, flamenco, or aerobic dancing. Or work out at your local gym.

Caution. Before you take up a competitive sport, get a full physical from your medical doctor. Competitive sports lead many to overexert themselves. For those with cardiovascular risk factors, overexertion can bring on a heart attack or stroke.

3. Be active throughout the day. Walk up stairs whenever possible. Avoid elevators to the lower floors. Take short, brisk walks on errands. Get out of your chair and move your body.

A SOCIETY ON THE BRINK, BUT YOU DO NOT HAVE TO FOLLOW

Insulin resistance, and its many terrible offspring, present a unique challenge to each of us as individuals, and to American society at large. These illnesses challenge us to examine some of our most accepted and cherished behaviors, including our food choices, exercise habits, and the ways we cope with stress. They also demand that we turn a more sophisticated and even skeptical eye at some of the powerful forces that shape our society and encourage us each day to consume more high-fat, high-protein, and highly processed foods—foods that virtually guarantee the kinds of epidemics that are destroying our lives today.

As you know, it isn't just diet alone, but the levels of stress in our lives, that encourages us to use food and escapist entertainment as analgesics against the pain of modern life. The sheer ubiquity of escapist entertainment, especially on television and computers, encourages us—and our children—to live ever more sedentary lives. A sedentary lifestyle, especially when it is joined by the modern diet, is a guarantee for elevated insulin, weight gain, high levels of inflammation, and an increased risk of major disease.

Our culture has presented all of us with a difficult choice. On the one hand, we are bombarded by images of lean and happy people eating high-fat, high-protein, and highly processed foods. The same media encourage us to stay riveted to the television—and while we're at it, we might as well have some snacks. The underlying message in this avalanche of advertising is that the only consequence of such behavior is joy. These images, the media tell us, are how we should behave in order to be considered "normal"—indeed, even a member of American society—in the twenty-first century.

On the other hand, we are informed by a convincing body of scientific evidence that the diet we are encouraged to eat, and the lifestyle we are urged to enjoy, is killing us. And the more we surrender to the current norms in diet and lifestyle, the greater our chances of becoming overweight and/or diabetic, and suffering any number of serious illnesses, including heart disease and cancer.

Once any of these degenerative diseases manifests, doctors work feverishly to do all they can to treat it. But as we know, there are limits to what medicine can do. Increasingly, truly effective treatment is seen as a partnership between doctor and patient, for the simple reason that there are things the patient can do that the doctor cannot, and those acts of self-healing can make all the world of difference.

Are we willing to be seduced by media images that try to convince us that we can indulge with impunity, or do we listen to the scientists who say that such behaviors are the basis for all the ravages we know as insulin resistance and its related disorders? Once we've answered that question, a second automatically arises: What are we willing to do to protect ourselves and those we love from these terrible epidemics?

· 12 ·

A Dietary Plan for Recovery

Following is an overview of a diet that will lower both your insulin levels and the inflammation in your body. It will strengthen your immune system, help protect you against diabetes, heart disease, cancer, and Alzheimer's disease.

After the general recommendations, we have provided a three-week menu plan. That is followed by more than fifty recipes for easy-to-prepare meals, all of which are insulin lowering.

GENERAL RECOMMENDATIONS:

Fish

Recommendations:

- East fish three or four times per week. Choose white fish, such as cod, flounder, haddock, halibut, scrod, and sole, as well as salmon. Avoid mackerel and swordfish, due to their mercury content.

Animal Products

Recommendations:

- Limit red meat and poultry to one four-ounce serving per day. Whenever possible, eat range-fed or organic beef, pork, chicken, and other animal foods to avoid excessive levels of hormones, antibiotics, and other substances that may affect how your cells and genes function.
- Eat only skim milk products and limit the amount of skim milk and skim milk products you consume. Avoid all whole milk products for their high levels of saturated fat. (As we showed in chapter 6, milk may drive up IGF-1 levels and may be associated with higher rates of breast, prostate, and ovarian cancers.)
- To facilitate the most rapid health promotion and recovery, eat two vegan meals per day, meaning two meals that contain no animal products, including meat, poultry, eggs, or dairy products.

Whole Grains

Recommendations:

- Eat a cooked whole grain at least once a day.
- Eat whole-grain products and high-quality pasta.

Whole grains include the following:

Brown Rice
Barley
Millet

Oats

Whole wheat and bulgur (whole-wheat bread is not a whole grain, but a processed grain.)

Quinoa

Amaranth

Buckwheat

Teff

Vegetables

Recommendations:

- Eat at least seven and preferably nine servings of vegetables per day. Serving size does not matter.
- Eat at least three servings of green and leafy vegetables per day.
- Eat at least one serving of a sweet vegetable per day, such as squash, sweet potato, yam, onion, carrot, parsnip, asparagus, or corn.

Recommended vegetables include the following:

Leafy Greens	Tubers	Roots
Asparagus	Artichokes	Burdock
Beet greens	String beans	Carrot
Carrot tops	Beets	Celery
Chinese cabbage	Broccoli	Daikon radish
Collard greens	Brussels sprouts	Icicle radish
Curly dock	Cabbage	Lotus root
Sprouts	Cucumber	Parsnip

(continued)

Leafy Greens	Tuber	Roots
Watercress	Green peas	Red radish
Dandelion greens	Snow peas	Rutabaga
Endive	Leeks	Salsify
Escarole	Shiitake mushrooms	Turnip
Kale	Onions	
Kohlrabi	Squashes	
Lamb's quarters	Acorn squash	
Lettuce	Butternut squash	
Mustard greens	Hakkaido pumpkin	
Parsley	Hubbard squash	
Scallion	Plantains	
	Pumpkin	
	Yellow squash	
	Zucchini	
	Yams or sweet potatoes	

Leaves and Stalks	Bulbs, Roots, and Tubers	Flowers, Fruits, and Seeds
Asparagus	Beet	Artichoke
Beet greens	Burdock	Broccoli
Brussels sprouts	Carrot	Cauliflower
Cabbage	Celery root	Cucumber
Carrot tops	Chicory root	Eggplant
Celery	Daikon radish	Green peas
Chard	Dandelion root	Mushrooms

Leaves and Stalks	Bulbs, Roots, and Tubers	Flowers, Fruits, and Seeds
Chinese cabbage	Garlic	Peppers
Collard greens	Jinenjo (mountain	Plantain
Curly dock	potato)	Pumpkin
Dandelion greens	Leek	Snow peas
Endive	Lotus root	String beans
Escarole	Onion	Sweet corn
Fennel	Parsnip	Tomato
Kale	Potato	Winter squash
Kohlrabi	Radishes	Yellow squash
Lamb's quarters	Rutabaga	Zucchini
Leek greens	Salsify	
Lettuce	Scallion	
Mustard greens	Shallot	
Parsley	Sweet potato	
Rhubarb	Turnip	
Spinach	Yams	
Sprouts		
Watercress		

Beans

    Recommendations:

- Eat at least five servings of beans per week.
- Eat tempeh and tofu occasionally.

The following beans are recommended:

Aduki

Black beans

Chickpeas

Lentils

Black-eyed peas

Kidney beans

Lima beans

Navy beans

Pinto beans

Soybeans

Fruit

Recommendations:

- Eat at least one piece of fruit daily.
- Eat fresh fruit.
- Avoid dried fruit. Dried fruit is rich in sugar and will drive up insulin levels.
- In general, make the majority of your fruits those that grow in your climate.

Nuts And Seeds

Recommendations:

- Eat a small handful of nuts three to five times per week.
- Add seeds—sunflower, sesame, and pumpkin—as a condiment on grains and vegetables.

Oils

Recommendation:

- Use plant oils to sauté vegetables five to seven times per week.

Recommended oils:

Olive

Sesame

Toasted sesame oil

**Foods to Minimize or Avoid for Maximum Health
and Rapid Weight Loss:**

Avoid all processed foods that contain the following:

- White flour products, such as those in rolls, muffins, pastries, and white bread
- White sugar, brown sugar, sugar in the "raw," turbinado sugar, aspartame, and other artificial sweeteners
- All artificial preservatives, colors, and flavors
- All foods that contain trans fats such as hydrogenated oils and margarines
- Corn oil

MENUS

Following are three weeks of breakfasts, lunches, and dinners. Recipes for every food listed in the menus are provided in the recipe section.

To cut down on preparation time, make a habit of cooking extra amounts for dinner so that you can bring leftovers to work the following day and eat them as lunch. Buy plastic containers to make it easier to bring lunch to work.

Every meal and recipe that we recommend is weight-reducing, insulin-lowering, and anti-inflammatory. Most of our readers will want to supplement their current diets with the menu plans and recipes we have provided. For those who want to lose weight and lower insulin levels quickly, we recommend that you follow the plan below for the full three-week period. In fact, you could subsist very happily on this diet for an even more extended period. We have deliberately left out foods that raise insulin and increase inflammation—and are common in the American diet.

Week One

SUNDAY

Breakfast—

    Oatmeal, walnuts, and raisins, garnished with flaxseeds and fruit

    Coffee or tea (herbal, black, or green)

Lunch—

    Hummus sandwich on whole-wheat bread or pita

    Water or tea

Dinner—

    Fish Soup

    Soba Noodle "Sushi" Roll

    Mixed leafy green salad (choose Salad Dressing)

    Daikon Pickles

    Mocha Custard

    Water or a glass of wine or beer

MONDAY
Breakfast—

    Scrambled Tofu

    Whole-grain toast

    Tea or water

Lunch—

    Soba Noodle "Sushi" Roll from last night

    Vegetables, from last night

    Tea or water

Dinner—

    Miso Soup

    Boiled Brown Rice

    Sweet Baked Beans

    Boiled Salad

    Vegetable "Chow Mein"

    Boiled Greens

    Water, tea

TUESDAY
Breakfast—

    Soft Barley

    Boiled Greens, from last night

    Miso Soup, from last night

    Herbal or black tea or water

Lunch—

    Boiled Brown Rice, from last night

    Sweet Baked Beans, from last night

Salad with dressing of your choice
Tea or water

Dinner—
Mung Bean Dahl
Millet with Vegetables
Sautéed Kale with onions
Waterless Parsnips
Apple Kanten

Wednesday
Breakfast—
Quinoa with Oats, sweetened with brown rice syrup, plus walnuts
and raisins

Lunch—
Tofu "Egg Salad" Sandwich
Tea or water

Dinner—
Mushroom-Barley Soup
Boiled Brown Rice
Aduki Beans with Squash
Greens Combo with Tahini Sauce
Boiled carrots
Water or tea

Thursday
Breakfast—
Mushroom-Barley Soup, from last night

Lunch—
    Boiled Brown Rice, from last night
    Aduki Beans with Squash, from last night
    Greens Combo, from last night
    Tea or water

Dinner—
    Red Lentil Soup
    Tabouli
    Fried Tempeh with Sauerkraut
    Baked Autumn Stew
    Boiled Greens
    Water or tea

Friday
Breakfast—
    Oatmeal cooked with raisins, sweetened with brown rice syrup,
        if desired, and topped with flax seeds

Lunch—
    Tempeh sandwich with mustard and cooked green vegetables
        on whole-wheat bread
    Water or tea

Dinner—
    Squash and Sweet Potato Soup
    Boiled Brown Rice
    Black Beans

Collards with Tofu Sauce
Kanten with fresh fruit
Water, tea, or a glass or beer or wine

SATURDAY
Breakfast—

Soft rice, made by adding water to last night's rice and simmer-
ing a few minutes in a saucepan. Sweeten with brown rice
syrup. Top with flaxseeds.

Lunch—

Boiled Brown Rice, from last night
Black Beans, from last night
Collards with Tofu Sauce, from last night

Dinner—

Miso Soup
Millet with Squash
Broiled Tofu
Mixed Greens
Carrot and Turnip Matchsticks

Week Two

SUNDAY

Breakfast—

    Millet with Squash, from last night

    Mixed Greens, from last night

    Coffee, tea, or water

Lunch—

    Greek Spirals

    Boiled Salad (make extra for dinner tonight.)

    Water or tea

Dinner—

    Miso Soup

    Pressure-Cooked Brown Rice

    Sweet Baked Beans

    Sautéed Greens

    Boiled Salad, from lunch

    Vegetable "Chow Mein"

MONDAY

Breakfast—

    Steel-cut oats cooked with raisins and walnuts, topped with flaxseeds.

Lunch—

    Squash and Sweet Potato Soup

    Whitefish Salad on whole-grain bread

    Cabbage and Cumin

Dinner—
> Watercress-Miso Soup
> Buckwheat and Bowties
> Sweet-and-Sour Vegetables
> Greens Stew with Chickpeas
> Rutabaga Pickle

TUESDAY
Breakfast—
> Soft Barley
> Greens, from last night
> Herbal tea, black tea, or water

Lunch—
> Miso Soup, from yesterday
> Greek Spirals
> Cucumber Salad

Dinner—
> French Onion Soup
> Brown Rice
> Boiled Autumn Stew
> Sautéed Greens
> Cooked fresh fruit
> Water, tea

WEDNESDAY
Breakfast—
> Soft rice, from last night (see Week One, Saturday breakfast)
> Autumn Stew, from last night

Lunch—

    Hummus sandwich on whole-wheat bread or pita

    Squash and Sweet Potato Soup

    Lovely Leeks

Dinner—

    Steamed Fish (cook extra for Thursday)

    Mixed Greens

    Roasted Potatoes

    Waterless Carrots

    Daikon Pickles

    Roasted Seeds and Raisins

THURSDAY

Breakfast—

    Bulgur and Oatmeal

Lunch—

    Whitefish Salad Sandwich (use fish from last night) or sardine
       sandwich

Dinner—

    Tofu and Millet Stew

    Brown Rice

    Mixed Greens

    Sweet Baked Beans

    Kanten, with apples

    Water, tea

Friday

Breakfast—

Tofu and Millet Stew, from last night

Mixed Greens, from last night

Lunch—

Fried Rice with Shrimp and Vegetables (use rice from last night)

Dinner—

Sukiyaki, over noodles of your choice

Salad with Dressing of your choice

Water, tea

Saturday

Breakfast—

Quinoa with Oats, and raisins, sweetened with brown rice syrup, if desired, topped with flaxseeds.

Lunch—

Leafy green sandwich, made by layering cooked leafy greens, sauerkraut, mustard, olive oil, soy sauce or any dressing you like, on a slice of whole-wheat bread.

Dinner—

Lentil Dahl (See "Mung Bean or Lentil Dahl" in recipes)

Buckwheat with Bowties

Waterless Rutabaga

Greens Rolls

Kanten with berries
Water, tea, beer, or wine

Week Three

SUNDAY
Breakfast—
   Oatmeal and raisins
   Greens Rolls, from last night
   Water, tea, coffee

Lunch—
   Lentil Dahl, from last night
   Buckwheat, from last night
   Cabbage and Cumin

Dinner—
   Watercress-Miso Soup
   Soba Noodle "Sushi" Rolls
   Aduki Beans with Squash
   Carrot and Turnip Matchsticks
   Mixed Greens
   Water, tea

MONDAY
Breakfast—
   Miso Soup, from last night
   Whole Oats
   Vegetables, from last night

Lunch—
    Hummus Sandwich on whole-wheat bread or pita

Dinner—
    Baked Salmon
    Vegetable "Chow Mein"
    Roasted Potatoes
    Mixed leafy salad
    Kanten, apricot juice with blueberries
    Water or tea

TUESDAY

Breakfast—
    Quinoa with Oats, walnuts, raisins
    Sautéed Greens

Lunch—
    Whitefish Salad Sandwich

Dinner—
    Black Bean Chili
    Tabouli
    Mixed Greens
    Waterless Parsnips
    Sweet-and-Sour Vegetables
    Water, tea

WEDNESDAY
Breakfast—
    Miso Soup
    Soft Barley
    Mixed Greens, from last night
    Water, tea

Lunch—
    Soba Noodle "Sushi" Rolls
    Sautéed Greens

Dinner—
    French Onion Soup
    Brown Rice
    Sweet Baked Beans
    Rutabaga Pickle
    Greens Combo with Tahini Sauce
    Water, tea

THURSDAY
Breakfast—
    Scrambled Tofu with whole-wheat toast
    Boiled Salad

Lunch—
    Fried Rice with Shrimp and Vegetables (use rice from last night)

Dinner—
- Millet with Vegetables
- Mung Bean Dahl
- Sautéed Greens
- Waterless Turnips
- Apple Kanten
- Water, tea

FRIDAY
Breakfast–
- Oatmeal cooked with raisins and walnuts, sweetened with brown rice syrup, if desired, and topped with flaxseeds

Lunch—
- Squash and Sweet Potato Soup
- Greek Spirals
- Cucumber Salad

Dinner—
- Steamed Fish
- Leafy green salad with salad dressing of your choice
- Roasted Potatoes
- Greens Rolls
- Vegetable "Chow Mein"
- Roasted Seeds and Raisins

SATURDAY
Breakfast—
- Quinoa with Oats, sweetened with brown rice syrup, if desired, and topped with sunflower seeds and raisins

Lunch—

Sardine sandwich with lettuce, tomato, and onion on whole-grain
bread

Dinner—

Squash and Sweet Potato Soup
Buckwheat and Bowties
Sweet-and-Sour Vegetables
Mixed Greens
Daikon Pickle

RECIPES

❖ Aduki Beans with Squash

2 cups aduki beans
1 winter squash, seeded and cubed (peeled if not organic)
1 stalk kombu seaweed (optional)
1 tablespoon tamari

Combine beans and kombu in 5 cups water and bring to boil. Turn
down to medium and cook for about $1^1/_2$ hours. Add squash and
tamari, and more water if necessary, and cook until squash is tender, approximately 15 minutes.

❖ Baked Autumn Stew

2 rutabagas, cut in large chunks
2 carrots, cut in large chunks
2 yams, diced
2 tablespoons tamari
2 tablespoons olive oil
6 tablespoons balsamic vinegar
$^1/_4$ cup brown rice syrup

Preheat oven to 375 degrees. Place veggies in baking pan. Combine tamari and olive oil, and coat vegetables with mixture. Drizzle combination of balsamic vinegar and rice syrup over the top. Cover and bake for $1^1/_2$ hours.

❖ Baked Salmon

1 tablespoon tamari
3 tablespoons olive oil
$^1/_2$ teaspoon dried dill
Juice from 1 lemon
$^1/_2$ onion, diced
$1^1/_2$ pounds salmon fillet

Combine tamari, olive oil, dill, lemon juice, and onion in a bowl. Place salmon in shallow baking dish, cover with sauce, and bake in preheated 350 degree oven for about $^1/_2$ hour, or until salmon becomes whitish and flakes easily.

❖ Baked Winter Squash

1 large butternut, acorn, or other winter squash

Wash and cut the squash in half. Take out the seeds. Place on a cookie sheet, cut side down. Bake in preheated oven at 350 to 375 degrees for about 1 hour. Test by pricking the center with a fork.

❖ Beans, Baked Sweet

2 cups pinto beans, soaked for a few hours
1 stalk kombu seaweed (optional)
$\frac{1}{2}$ cup miso
$\frac{1}{2}$ cup apple butter
1 tablespoon prepared mustard

Boil beans with kombu in 2 quarts water for 2 hours. (If you add the kombu, it will help the beans to soften and make them more digestible.) Turn flame down to simmer, and add other ingredients. If you like the beans more salty, add more miso. If you like a sweeter taste, add more apple butter. Transfer to a baking dish and bake at 350 degrees until beans have a nice sauce, but aren't too watery.

❖ Beet Salad

4 beets
$\frac{1}{4}$ cup olive oil
2 tablespoons balsamic vinegar

Touch of prepared mustard
Salt and pepper, to taste
1 red onion, sliced

Trim and wash the beets. Bring whole beets to a boil in enough water
to cover. Cook for about 25 minutes, or until soft. Drain beets and
allow to cool. Peel and slice beets. Add oil, vinegar, mustard, salt and
pepper, and red onion. Marinate for a few hours in the refrigerator.

✣ Black Beans

2 cups black beans, soaked for a few hours
1 onion, chopped
1 clove garlic, minced
1 tablespoon ground cumin
1 tablespoon ground coriander
1 teaspoon sea salt
Pinch of cayenne

Place beans in 6 cups water and bring to a boil. Cook on medium
flame for $1\frac{1}{2}$ hours. Add other ingredients and simmer for 30 minutes more, or until beans are soft.

✣ Black Bean Chili

2 cups black beans, soaked for a few hours
1 onion, diced
1 red or green bell pepper, seeded and diced
2 tomatoes, diced

2 cloves garlic, minced

3 tablespoons tamari

2 teaspoons umeboshi vinegar

1 tablespoon chili powder

Chopped parsley

Place beans in 6 cups water and bring to a boil. Cook on medium flame for 1^1/$_2$ hours. Add onion, pepper, tomatoes, garlic, tamari, vinegar, and chili powder. Cook together another half hour. Garnish with chopped parsley.

❖ Boiled Autumn Stew

2 parsnips, cut in large chunks

2 carrots, cut in large chunks

1 small winter squash, seeded and cut in large chunks (peeled if not organic)

^{1}/$_2$ teaspoon sea salt

Place vegetables and salt in a pot and cover with ^{1}/$_2$ inch water. Bring to a boil. Simmer, covered, for 1 hour or until vegetables are soft.

❖ Boiled Brown Rice

1 cup brown rice

Sea salt

Combine rice and salt with 3 cups water in a pot and bring to a boil. Simmer for 1 hour.

✤ Boiled Greens

Any green leafy vegetables, trimmed

Bring a pot of water to a boil. Add greens and boil for 3 to 5 minutes. Drain, cool, and slice. Serve seasoned with olive oil, tamari, lemon juice, or your favorite dressing.

✤ Boiled Salad

1 head cabbage, cored and cut in chunks
2 turnips, cut in chunks
1 tablespoon tahini, diluted with a little water
2 tablespoons tamari
Juice from 1 orange
Juice from 1 lemon

Bring a pot of water to a boil. Drop in cabbage chunks. Remove after a few minutes, so that cabbage is still crisp. Drop turnips into the water for a few minutes and remove when turnips are still crisp. Mix the tahini and tamari in a small pot and cook on low flame for a minute or two. Remove from heat and add orange and lemon juice. Pour over the vegetables.

❖ Brown Rice Balls

Brown rice (works best when rice is pressure-cooked)
Sushi nori seaweed
Umeboshi paste, other kind of pickle, or olives

Wet your hands with cold, salted water and form rice into a small ball. Take a little umeboshi paste and stick it into the middle of the rice ball with your finger. Wrap nori seaweed around the rice ball and seal closed.

❖ Broiled Tofu

1 cake tofu
2 tablespoons tamari
2 teaspoons grated ginger

Heat the broiler. Place tofu on a broiler pan. Mix tamari and ginger together and sprinkle over tofu. Broil tofu on each side until slightly brown. Keep an eye on this, as it can burn quickly.

❖ Buckwheat and Bowties

1 cup buckwheat groats
1 onion, diced
$^1/_2$ celery stalk, diced
Sesame oil
A handful of cooked bowtie noodles

Tamari, to taste
Umeboshi vinegar, to taste
Sauerkraut, as much as desired
Parsley

Bring 3 cups water to a boil and add buckwheat. Cook for about 20 minutes, or until groats are soft. In a frying pan, sauté onion and celery in a little sesame oil and add cooked buckwheat, noodles, and seasonings. Toss with sauerkraut and parsley.

❖ Cabbage and Cumin

1   head cabbage, cored and chopped small
1   tablespoon sea salt
1   tablespoon ground cumin
2   tablespoons olive oil

Sauté the cabbage, salt, and cumin in oil in a frying pan for 10 minutes. Add a little water if necessary, cover, and steam for 5 minutes.

❖ Carrot and Turnip Matchsticks

2   cups turnip matchsticks
2   cups carrot matchsticks
2   teaspoons sesame oil
Sprinkle of sea salt

Place turnips and carrots into frying pan coated with sesame oil. Sprinkle with sea salt, and sauté a few minutes.

❖ Collards with Tofu Sauce

2 bunches of collard greens, heavy stems trimmed
1 cake soft tofu
1 teaspoon grated ginger
2 tablespoons white miso
2 tablespoons umeboshi vinegar

Steam collards whole for about 5 minutes. Drain, and slice into thin pieces.

Puree together tofu, ginger, $1/4$ cup water, miso, and vinegar. Add to collards.

❖ Cucumber Salad

4 cucumbers, sliced thin
1 teaspoon sea salt
1 teaspoon tamari
1 teaspoon toasted sesame oil
1 teaspoon brown rice vinegar
3 tablespoons toasted sesame seeds

Place cucumber and salt in a colander or a bowl, and cover with a plate and place a weight on top. Press for 1 hour or more. Drain the liquid. Rinse off the salt. Add tamari, sesame oil, and vinegar. Toss to combine. Garnish with toasted sesame seeds.

❖ Daikon Pickles

1 cup diced or thinly sliced daikon
$\frac{1}{2}$ cup tamari
$\frac{1}{4}$ cup lemon juice

Place daikon in a jar. Add tamari and lemon juice, plus enough water to make sure all the daikon pieces are covered. Allow to marinate overnight.

❖ Fish Soup

$\frac{3}{4}$ pound firm-fleshed white fish
2 cups diced onion
1 cup diced carrots
1 cup diced cabbage
2 tablespoons tamari
Grated ginger, to taste
Scallions, sliced thin

Rinse the fish and cut into small pieces. Combine fish, vegetables, tamari, and 2 quarts water in a pot. Cover and simmer over low heat for about 25 minutes. Add grated ginger and sliced scallions.

❖ French Onion Soup

5 onions, sliced
Sesame oil

Touch of salt
Tamari, to taste
Chopped parsley

Sauté onions in a little sesame oil in a large pot with a touch of salt. Cover and simmer for at least ½ hour. Add 5 cups water, reduce heat, and cook another ½ hour. Season with tamari to taste and simmer 5 minutes more. Garnish with parsley.

❧ Fried Rice with Shrimp and Vegetables

1 tablespoon olive oil
1 clove garlic, minced
1 cup broccoli florets
1 cup thinly sliced carrots
1 cup cooked rice
1 cup thinly sliced scallions
¼ pound shrimp, cooked and diced
1 tablespoon tamari
¼ teaspoon umeboshi vinegar
1 teaspoon grated ginger
1 sheet sushi nori seaweed, broken up in small pieces

Heat oil in a skillet and add garlic, broccoli, and carrots and stir for 10 seconds. Cover and cook a few minutes longer if broccoli is not yet tender. Add rice, scallions, shrimp, tamari, vinegar, ginger, and sushi nori. Stir together until everything is well mixed and rice is coated with sauce.

❖ Fried Tempeh with Sauerkraut

1 package tempeh, any flavor
Tamari, to taste
Sesame oil
Sauerkraut (store-bought organic)

Cook tempeh in one cup of water with tamari for $1/2$ hour. (You can skip this step and just fry it, but I have found cooking it first makes it more digestible.) Drain and pat dry. Fry the tempeh in sesame oil until golden brown on each side. Drain on paper towels and season with tamari to taste. Arrange in bowl on top of sauerkraut.

❖ Greek Spirals

6 cups whole-wheat spiral noodles
1 onion, diced
10 button mushrooms, wiped clean and diced
10 cups fresh spinach, washed, dried, and chopped small
5 sun-dried tomatoes, soaked for 20 minutes and diced
1 teaspoon minced garlic
3 tablespoons olive oil
Tamari, to taste
Handful of pine nuts

Cook noodles. Drain and rinse thoroughly with cold water. In a large frying pan, sauté onion, mushrooms, spinach, tomatoes, and garlic in oil and tamari. When vegetables are soft, mix in noodles and pine nuts.

❖ Greens Combo with Tahini Sauce

    1 bunch kale, heavy stems trimmed
    1 bunch mustard greens, heavy stems trimmed
    1 head Chinese cabbage
    1 bunch broccoli, separated into stalks

Tahini sauce:
    2 tablespoon tahini
    3 tablespoons umeboshi paste
    2 tablespoons grated onion

Bring a large pot of water to a boil. Cook greens, uncut, for five to ten minutes. Drain, cool, and slice.

Combine sauce ingredients with $\frac{1}{4}$ cup water in a pot. Cook over low flame for a few minutes. Serve over greens combo.

❖ Greens Stew with Chickpeas

    2 tablespoons olive oil
    4 bunches of scallions, diced
    2 cloves garlic, minced
    2 tablespoons whole-wheat flour
    5 cups water
    $\frac{1}{4}$ teaspoon sea salt

2 cups garbanzo beans, cooked
1 cup kale, chopped
1 cup collard greens, chopped
1 cup mustard greens, chopped
1 cup arugula, chopped
1 cup broccoli, chopped

In a large pot, heat oil and sauté scallions and garlic until everything is soft. Add flour and cook a few minutes longer. Slowly add water and continue to stir. Add salt. Mixture will begin to thicken. Next add beans and greens. Cover and simmer for fifteen minutes or until greens are soft.

✣ Greens Rolls

3 carrots sticks
6 large Chinese cabbage leaves
1 bunch collard greens, heavy
1 bunch arugula
Toasted sesame oil
Umeboshi vinegar

Bring a pot of water to a boil. Boil each vegetable separately until tender. Drain and cool each separately. Place 1 to 3 collard green leaves depending on size of leaf on a bamboo rolling mat. Top with a few Chinese cabbage leaves, some arugula, and a carrot stick. Roll the collard green leaves in the mat, as you would if you were making sushi. Squeeze gently to remove excess water and seal the roll. Slice into 1-inch rounds and sit upright on serving platter. Make a sauce with equal parts toasted sesame oil and umeboshi vinegar. Drizzle over the rolls.

✣ Hummus

2 cups cooked and drained chickpeas
¼ cup lemon juice
4 cloves garlic
3 tablespoons tahini
1 teaspoon salt

Puree everything together in a food processor or blender. Add water to desired consistency. Enjoy with crackers, use as a vegetable dip, or make a sandwich.

✣ Kanten

This is apple kanten, but any fruit juice or fruits can be substituted.

4 cups apple juice
6 tablespoons agar flakes
Sprinkle of sea salt
3 medium apples, cored and sliced

Place juice, agar, salt, and 2 cups water in a pot. Bring to a simmer and cook 5 minutes, stirring constantly. Add apples and simmer for another 5 minutes, stirring constantly. Pour into a mold or several cups, and allow to chill until set. Serve cold.

❖ Lovely Leeks

5 or 6 leeks, cut into 1-inch slices (white and light green only)
   and washed
1 carrot, diced
1 turnip, diced
1 tablespoon olive oil
1 teaspoon tamari
2 teaspoons brown rice syrup
1 tablespoon prepared mustard
1 teaspoon brown rice vinegar

Cook leeks, carrot, and turnip in oil in a frying pan on low flame, covered, for about 25 minutes. Remove cover and cook until there is no remaining liquid. Put tamari, rice syrup, mustard, and vinegar in a covered jar and shake. Stir into the vegetables.

❖ Millet with Vegetables

2 cups millet
1 onion, chopped
1 carrot,
½ head cauliflower, chopped
Sea salt, to taste

Combine ingredients in a pot with 8 cups water and bring to boil. Simmer 1 hour.

✤ Millet with Squash

2 cups millet
¼ winter squash, seeded and cubed (peel if not organic)
Sea salt, to taste

Combine ingredients in a pot with 8 cups of water and bring to a boil. Simmer 1 hour.

✤ Miso Soup

Any three vegetables can be used.

1 stalk kombu (optional)
Handful of bonito flakes (optional)
3 dried shiitake mushrooms, soaked and sliced in half (optional)
1 onion, diced
½ head small cabbage, cored and diced
2 tablespoons miso
Grated ginger, to taste

Bring 6 cups water to a boil. Add kombu, bonito flakes, and shiitake mushrooms, if using. Add onion and cabbage, cover, and simmer and until vegetables are soft. Remove 1 cup of stock and stir in miso. Return to pot and simmer (don't boil) for 10 minutes. Turn off flame and add grated ginger. Remove kombu before serving.

✤ Mixed Greens

2 bunches scallions, sliced
1 tablespoon olive oil
4 cloves garlic, minced
1 tablespoon whole-wheat flour
Sprinkle of sea salt
Sprinkle of pepper
4 cups chopped kale, collards, watercress, Chinese cabbage, and/
 or other greens
Umeboshi vinegar and tamari, to taste

Sauté scallions and garlic in olive oil until soft. Stir in flour and coat the scallions. Add 2 cups water, salt, and pepper and simmer a few minutes, or until slightly thick. Add greens and cook for at least 15 minutes. Season with vinegar and tamari.

✤ Mocha Custard

1 tablespoon tahini
4 cups apple juice
3 tablespoons agar agar flakes
$\frac{1}{8}$ teaspoons sea salt
3 tablespoons kuzu
$1\frac{1}{2}$ tablespoons grain coffee (coffee substitute)
$\frac{1}{8}$ teaspoon cinnamon
$\frac{1}{2}$ teaspoon vanilla extract

Dilute the tahini, agar agar flakes, and salt in 3 cups of juice. Place in a saucepan and bring to a boil, stirring constantly. Lower flame. Stir and simmer for five more minutes. Turn off flame and let sit. Meanwhile, dilute kuzu and grain coffee in $1/2$ cup of juice. Add to tahini-agar agar mixture. Then add $1/2$ cup of juice, cinnamon, and vanilla and bring to a boil, stirring constantly so the kuzu doesn't clump. Allow to cool at room temperature.

❖ Mung Bean or Lentil Dahl

1 cup dried mung beans or lentils
1 strip kombu seaweed
2 cloves garlic, minced
1 teaspoon ground cumin
1 teaspoon ground turmeric
Sprinkle of black pepper
$1/2$ head cauliflower, broken into florets
1 onion, diced
Olive oil
1 tablespoon miso, or to taste
1 scallion, chopped

Soak mung beans for a few hours. (Lentils don't have to be soaked.) Add kombu and water to cover and boil for $1^1/2$ hours (mung beans) or 1 hour (lentils). Sauté all the other ingredients, except miso and scallions in oil. Add to the beans. Cook another $1/2$ hour until everything is mushy. Turn flame to low, stir in miso, and cook another 10 minutes. Garnish with scallions.

❖ Mushroom-Barley Soup

3 dried shiitake mushrooms, soaked and diced
$\frac{1}{2}$ cup pearled barley
1 onion, diced
2 carrots, diced
7 leaves Chinese cabbage, cut in big squares
$\frac{1}{2}$ cup miso
1 scallion, sliced
Grated ginger, for garnish

Put shiitakes and barley in a pot and and add 5 cups water. Bring to a boil. Simmer 20 minutes. Add onion, carrots, and cabbage and simmer at least 1 hour. Mix in miso. Simmer 10 minutes more. Garnish with sliced scallions and grated ginger.

❖ Pressure-Cooked Brown Rice

1 cup brown rice
Sprinkle of sea salt

Place rice, 3 cups water, and salt in pressure cooker. Bring to pressure. Turn down to low and cook for about 45 minutes.

❖ Oatmeal and Bulgur

1 cup bulgur
1 cup rolled oats
1 pinch sea salt

Combine all ingredients in a saucepan with 4 cups water and bring to boil. Simmer 30 to 40 minutes.

❖ Quinoa with Oats

1 cup quinoa, soaked for 20 minutes
1 cup rolled oats
Sea salt

Combine all ingredients in a saucepan with 3 cups water and bring to a boil. Simmer 30 minutes.

❖ Red Lentil Soup

1 cup lentils
1 onion, diced
2 carrots, diced
2 beets, peeled and diced
¼ cup miso (dark miso is nice in this soup)
Chopped parsley

Put lentils and vegetables in pot with 6 cups water and bring to a boil. Simmer for at least 1 hour. Working carefully in batches, blend soup in blender and return to the pot. Cream miso in small bowl with a little bit of the soup, and return to pot. Simmer another 10 minutes. Garnish with parsley.

✤ Roasted Potatoes

1 pound bag small yellow or red potatoes, well scrubbed
Olive oil
Salt and pepper

Coat potatoes generously with olive oil in a baking pan. Sprinkle them with salt and pepper and bake at 350 degrees for $1^{1}/_{2}$ hours, or until tender.

✤ Roasted Seeds and Raisins

Roast sunflower seeds and raisins together in a frying pan, stirring occasionally until seeds get slightly brown. Drizzle brown rice syrup on top, if a sweeter taste is desired.

✤ Rutabaga Pickle

1 rutabaga, cut up in small pieces
Tamari

Cover rutabaga with tamari and refrigerate for at least 24 hours. If pickle is too salty, rinse with cold water.

❖ Salad Dressings

MUSTARD DRESSING
 6 tablespoons lemon juice
 ¼ cup tamari
 2 teaspoons prepared mustard
 3 tablespoons olive oil

Place ingredients in a jar with 6 tablespoons water and shake until blended.

ORANGE-MISO DRESSING
 2 teaspoons white miso
 1 teaspoon toasted sesame oil
 ¼ cup orange juice

Cream the miso with the sesame oil and orange juice in a small bowl.

SESAME-LEMON DRESSING
 2 tablespoons sesame oil
 2 tablespoons lemon juice
 1 tablespoon brown rice vinegar
 2 tablespoons tamari

Put all ingredients in a covered jar with ½ cup water and shake until well mixed.

❖ Sautéed Greens

1 bunch greens (kale, collard, arugula, mustard greens), heavy
   stems trimmed
1 large onion, diced
1 clove garlic
1 tablespoon olive oil or sesame oil
Tamari, to taste

Boil a pot of water and add greens (no need to slice them up). Cook
for 1 to 3 minutes. Drain and cut into strips. Meanwhile, sauté
onion and garlic in oil in a frying pan. Throw in the greens and
add a little tamari.

❖ Soba Noodle "Sushi" Roll

1 package soba noodles
1 tablespoon toasted sesame oil
1 tablespoon regular sesame oil
2 tablespoons tamari
2 tablespoons brown rice vinegar
1½ teaspoons grated ginger
1½ teaspoons grated garlic
1 package nori

Cook noodles according to package directions. Drain but don't
rinse. Sauté noodles in sesame oils. Off the heat add tamari, vinegar, ginger, and garlic, and toss to combine. Allow noodles to cool.

Place sushi nori on bamboo mat (for rolling) and put some soba noodles on the nori, leaving about ¼ inch at the bottom of the nori and a few inches at the top. Using the mat, roll up nori while continually pushing the noodles closer together. Take a wet, sharp knife and cut the roll into 8 even pieces.

✤ Soft Barley

1 cup barley
Pinch of sea salt

Combine barley and salt with 5 cups water in a pot and bring to a boil. Simmer 1½ hours. Sweeten with brown rice syrup, if desired. Garnish with sunflower seeds, flaxseeds, raisins.

✤ Squash and Sweet Potato Soup

8 cups peeled, seeded, and cubed winter squash
1 large sweet potato, cubed
2 tablespoons barley miso

Cut the skin off the squash and remove the seeds. Place squash, sweet potato, and 3 cups water in a pot. Bring to a boil and simmer for about 1 hour, or until the vegetables are soft. Add miso and simmer on low for 5 minutes. For a creamy consistency, puree in batches in a blender.

❖ Steamed Fish

2 pounds white fish fillets

3 tablespoons tamari

1 tablespoon toasted sesame oil

1 tablespoon brown rice syrup

Grated ginger, to taste

Grated garlic, to taste

$\frac{1}{2}$ red pepper, diced

$\frac{1}{2}$ green pepper, diced

Place fish on a plate over boiling water in steamer. Mix other ingredients together and pour over fish. Let steam about 5 minutes, depending on thickness of fish, or until fish flakes.

❖ Sukiyaki

1 onion, sliced

6 cups broccoli florets

1 large carrot, sliced

$\frac{1}{2}$ head cabbage, cored and sliced

$\frac{1}{2}$ butternut squash, sliced (peeled if not organic)

Sprinkle of sea salt

Kale leaves, heavy stems trimmed, sliced

$\frac{1}{3}$ cup sake or mirin

3 tablespoons tamari

Grated ginger, to taste

$\frac{1}{2}$ cake tofu, cubed

Place onion, broccoli, carrot, cabbage, and squash in a frying pan. Add water to cover and sprinkle with salt. Bring to a boil. Reduce to simmer and cook 10 minutes, or until vegetables are tender. Add kale and cook another 3 minutes, covered. Combine sake, tamari, and ginger and pour over vegetables. Add tofu. Simmer a few minutes longer.

❖ Sweet-and-Sour Vegetables

3 leeks, cut into slices (white and light green only) and washed
1 carrot, sliced
1 turnip, halved and sliced
Olive oil
1 teaspoon tamari
2 teaspoons brown rice syrup
1 tablespoon prepared mustard
1 teaspoon brown rice vinegar

Sauté leeks, carrot, and turnip with oil and tamari for 25 minutes, uncovered. Add a little water, if needed. Cook until everything is soft and there is no liquid left. Put rice syrup, mustard, and vinegar in a jar and shake. Stir into veggies.

❖ Tabouli

1 cup bulgur wheat
Salt, to taste
1 cup chopped parsley
1 onion, diced

1 tomato, diced
Juice of 1 lemon
1 tablespoon olive oil
Fresh or dried mint, to taste

Bring 2 cups water to a boil. Add bulgur and salt. Cook on low, covered, for 25 minutes. Turn off flame, and toss the rest of the ingredients with bulgur. Cool.

❖ Tofu "Egg Salad" Sandwich

1 cake tofu
¼ cup Nayonnaise (tofu mayonnaise)
½ cup chopped celery
¼ cup chopped scallion
Sprinkle of salt

Simmer tofu in water for 15 minutes. Drain, crumble into bowl, squeeze out and discard any additional liquid, and add the other ingredients. Mash and mix them all together. Serve on whole-grain bread with lettuce and sliced red onion.

❖ Tofu and Millet Stew

1 cup millet
½ cake tofu, cubed
2 carrots, sliced
1 stalk celery, sliced
Pinch of sea salt

Combine all ingredients in a pot with 6 cups water. Bring to a boil. Cover and cook over low heat for about 1 hour.

❖ Tofu, Scrambled

1 onion, chopped
1 clove garlic, minced
Olive oil
1 cake tofu
1 tablespoon curry powder
1 tablespoon ground turmeric

Sauté onion and garlic in oil until transparent. Crumble tofu and add along with curry powder and turmeric. Cover and simmer for about 15 minutes.

❖ Vegetable "Chow Mein"

1 onion, sliced
2 carrots, sliced
½ package button mushrooms, wiped clean and sliced
5 cups broccoli florets
Touch of tamari
1 bag mung bean sprouts
2 scallions, sliced lengthwise

SAUCE
1 teaspoon mirin
1 tablespoon tamari

$^1/_2$ cup water

2 tablespoons kuzu

2 teaspoons grated ginger

Put onion, carrots, mushrooms, broccoli, and tamari in wok or frying pan. Stir continually for 5 minutes, or until vegetables get soft but crispy. Add sprouts and scallions. Simmer a few minutes more.

Combine sauce ingredients in a separate bowl and then stir into vegetables.

❖ Watercress-Miso Soup

1 bunch watercress, washed and chopped (including stems)

4 teaspoons miso, or to taste

Bring 5 cups water to a boil. Add watercress to boiling water and cook for a minute or two. Turn fire to low. Remove some of the broth and dilute miso with it in a small bowl. Return the miso mixture to the pot and simmer on low for 10 minutes longer.

❖ Waterless Vegetables

These vegetables cook in their own juices and need very little seasoning. This is a recipe for waterless parsnips, but use any root vegetable or combo that you want. Generally, you should cut vegetables in chunks during the fall and winter, and cut more matchsticks during the spring and summer months.

3 parsnips, cut into chunks
1 onion, cut into chunks
Touch of sea salt

Place parsnips and onion in a heavy pot or cast-iron skillet. Add just enough water to almost cover the vegetables, a touch of salt, and bring to a boil. Lower the flame to simmer and cook until the vegetables are tender and water is almost gone, about $\frac{1}{2}$ hour. If vegetables aren't yet cooked, and you are running low on water, just add a little bit more.

❖ Whitefish Salad Sandwich

1 pound white fish fillets
1 cup diced celery
1 cup sliced scallions
1 tablespoon Nayonnaise (tofu mayonnaise)

Steam fish over a small amount of water until tender. Drain and cool. Mix thoroughly with other ingredients. Serve on whole-grain rolls with lettuce and sliced tomatoes.

❖ Whole Oats

1 cup whole oats
Sea salt

Combine oats and salt in a pot with 6 cups water and bring to a boil. Simmer 2 to 3 hours.

Resources for Purchasing
Uncommon Foods Used in Our Recipes

———————————•———————————

Most of the foods listed in the dietary recommendations and recipes can be purchased at your local supermarket or natural foods store, or at the larger natural foods supermarket chains, such as Whole Foods Market or Wild Oats Supermarket.

You can also purchase natural foods through a wide array of mail-order supermarkets. Information for some of those markets is provided below.

Eden Foods
Full line of natural and organic foods
701 Tecumseh Road
Clinton, Michigan 49236
888-441-3336
888-424-3336
www.edenfoods.com

Diamond Organics
*Organic produce, grains, fruits, and other foods shipped
fresh overnight (guaranteed)*
Kitchen equipment
P.O. Box 2159
Freedom, California 95019
888-674-2642
www.diamondorganics.com

Jaffe Brothers
Organic fruits and nuts
28560 Lilac Road
Valley Center, California 92082
760-749-1133 (tel.)
760-749-1282 (fax.)
www.organicfruitsandnuts.com

Gold Mine Natural Food Co.
Full line of organic and natural foods
7805 Arjons Drive
San Diego, California 92126
800-475-3663
www.goldminenaturalfood.com

Natural Lifestyle
Full line of organic and natural foods
16 Lookout Drive
Asheville, North Carolina 28804
800-752-2772
www.natural-lifestyle.com

Miracle Exclusives
Kitchen equipment
64 Seaview Boulevard
Port Washington, New York 11050
800-645-6360
www.miracleexclusives.com

Bibliography

———•———

Adam, Tanja C. and Elissa S. Epel. "Stress, eating and the reward system." *Physiology and Behavior* 91:4 (July 24, 2007): 449–58.

Araghi-Niknam, Mohsen and S. Hossein Fatemi. "Levels of Bcl-2 and P53 Are Altered in Superior Frontal and Cerebellar Cortices of Autistic Subjects." *Cellular and Molecular Neurobiology* 23:6 (December 2003): 945–952.

Altfas, Jules R. "Prevalence of attention deficit/hyperactivity disorder among adults in obesity treatment." *BMC Psychiatry* 2:9 (September 13, 2002).

Augustin, L. S. A.; L. Dal Maso, C. La Vecchia, M. Parpinel, E. Negri, S. Vaccarella, C.W.C. Kendall, D.J.A. Jenkins, and S. Franceschi. "Dietary glycemic index and glycemic load, and breast cancer risk: A case-control study." *Annals of Oncology* 12:11 (November 2001): 1533–38.

Barnard, R. J., W. J. Aronson, C. N. Tymchuk, and T. H. Ngo. "Prostate cancer: another aspect of the insulin-resistance syndrome?" *Obesity Reviews* 3:4 (2002): 303–8.

Bazar, Kimberly A., Anthony J. Yun, Patrick Y. Lee, Stephanie M. Daniel, and John D. Doux. "Obesity and ADHD may represent different manifestations of a common environmental oversampling syndrome: a model for revealing mechanistic overlap among cognitive, metabolic, and inflammatory disorders." *Medical Hypotheses* 6:2 (2006): 263–69

Ballard-Barbash, Rachel, Arthur Schatzkin, Christine L. Carter, William B. Kannel, Bernard E. Kreger, Ralph B. D'Agostino, Greta L. Splansky, Keaven M. Anderson, and William E. Helsel. "Body Fate Distribution and Breast Cancer in the Framingham Study." *Journal of the National Cancer Institute* 82 (1990): 286–90.

Bråkenhielm, Ebba, Niina Veitonmäki, Renhai Cao, Shinji Kihara, Yuji Matsuzawa, Boris Zhivotovsky, Tohru Funahashi, and Yihai Cao. "Adiponectin-induced antiangiogenesis and antitumor activity involve caspase-mediated endothelial cell apoptosis." *Proceedings of the National Academy of Sciences* 101:8 (February 24, 2004): 2476–81.

Bray, George A., Jennifer C. Lovejoy, Steven R. Smith, James P. DeLany, Michael Lefevre, Daniel Hwang, Donna H. Ryan, and David A. York. "The Influence of Different Fats and Fatty Acids on Obesity, Insulin Resistance and Inflammation." *Journal of Nutrition* 132 (September 2002): 2488–91.

Calle, Eugenia E., Carmen Rodriguez, Kimberly Walker-Thurmond, and Michael J. Thun. "Overweight, Obesity, and Mortality from Cancer in a Prospectively Studied Cohort of U.S. Adults." *New England Journal of Medicine* 348 (April 24, 2003): 1625–38.

Cha, Ming C. and Peter J. H. Jones. "Dietary fat type and energy restriction interactively influence plasma leptin concentration in rats." *Journal of Lipid Research* 39 (August 1998): 1655–60.

Craft, Suzanne. "Insulin resistance syndrome and Alzheimer's disease: Age- and obesity-related effects on memory, amyloid, and inflammation." *Neurobiology of Aging* 26:1 (December 2005): 65–69.

Eaton, S. Boyd and Melvin Konner. "Paleolithic Nutrition." *New England Journal of Medicine* 312 (1985): 283–89.

Friedrich, M. J. "Insulin Effects Weigh Heavy on the Brain." *Journal of the American Medical Association* 296 (October 11, 2006): 1717–18.

Grady, Denise. "Link Between Diabetes and Alzheimer's Deepens." *New York Times*. July 17, 2006.

Herbert, J. R., T. H. Hurley, and Y. Ma. "The effect of dietary exposure on recurrence and mortality in early stage breast cancer." *Breast Cancer Research and Treatment* 51 (September 1998): 17–28.

Larson, Eric B.; Li Wang, James D. Bowen, Wayne C. McCormick, Linda Teri, Paul Crane, and Walter Kukull. "Exercise Is Associated with Reduced Risk for Incident Dementia among Persons 65 Years of Age and Older." *Annals of Internal Medicine* 144:2 (January 2006): 73–81.

Lewis, Thomas, Fari Amini, and Richard Lannon. *A General Theory of Love.* Vintage Books, 2000.

Lee, Woo Je,; Kee-Ho Song, Eun Hee Koh, Jong Chul Won, Hyoun Sik Kim, Hye-Sun Park, Min-Seon Kim, Seung-Whan Kim, Ki-Up Lee, and Joong-Yeol Park. "α-Lipoic acid increases insulin sensitivity by activating AMPK in skeletal muscle." *Biochemical and Biophysical Research Communications* 332:3 (July 2005): 885–91.

Liu, Simin,; Yiqing Song, Earl S. Ford, JoAnn E. Manson, Julie E. Buring, and Paul M. Ridker. "Dietary Calcium, Vitamin D, and the Prevalence of Metabolic Syndrome in Middle-Aged and Older U.S. Women." *Diabetes Care* 28:12 (December 2005): 2926–32.

Matarese, Giuseppe, Veronica Sanna, Robert I. Lechler, Nora Sarvetnick, Silvia Fontana, Serafino Zappacosta, and Antonio La Cava. "Leptin accelerates autoimmune diabetes in female NOD mice." *Diabetes* 51:5 (May 2002): 1356–61.

Miyoshi, Yasuo, Tohru Funahashi, Shinji Kihara, Tesuya Taguchi, Yasuhiro Tamaki, Yuji Matsuzawa, and Shinzaburo Noguchi. "Association of Serum Adiponectin Levels with Breast Cancer Risk." *Clinical Cancer Research* 9 (November 15, 2003): 5699–5704.

O'Dea, Kerin. "Obesity and Diabetes in the 'Land of Milk and Honey.' " *Diabetes/Metabolism Reviews* 8:4 (1992): 373–88.

O'Leary, Valerie B., Christine M. Marchetti, Raj K. Krishnan, Bradley P. Stetzer, Frank Gonzalez, and John P. Kirwan. "Exercise-induced reversal of insulin resistance in obese elderly is associated with reduced visceral fat." *Journal of Applied Physiology,* 101:8 (December 22, 2005): 76–81.

Panza F., V. Solfrizzi, A. M. Colacicco, A. D'Introno, C. Capurso, F. Torres, A. Del Parigi, S. Capurso, and A. Capurso. "Mediterranean diet and cognitive decline." *Public Health Nutrition* 7:7 (October 2004): 959–63.

Pritikin, Robert. *The Pritikin Principle: The Calorie Density Solution.* Des Moines, Iowa: Time-Life Books, 2000.

Pritikin, Robert. *The Pritikin Weight Loss Breakthrough.* New York: Dutton Books, 1998.

Renehan, Andrew G., Margaret Tyson, Matthias Egger, Richard F. Heller, and Marcel Zwahlen. "Body-mass index and incidence of cancer: a systematic review and meta-analysis of prospective observational studies." *The Lancet* 371:9612 (February 2008): 569–78

Saari, Kaisa M., Sari M. Lindeman, Kaisa M. Viilo, Matti K. Isohanni, Marjo-Riita Järvelin, Liisa H. Laurén, Markku J. Savolainen, and Hannu J. Koponen. "A 4-Fold Risk of Metabolic Syndrome in Patients With Schizophrenia: The Northern Finland 1966 Birth Cohort Study." *Journal of Clinical Psychiatry* 66:5 (May 2005).

Saxe, Gordon A., Cheryl L. Rock, Max S. Wicha, and David Schottenfeld. "Diet and risk for breast cancer recurrence and survival." *Breast Cancer Treatment,* 53:3 (February 1999): 241–53.

Schrauwen, Patrick and Klaas R. Westerterp. "The role of high-fat diets and physical activity in the regulation of body weight." *British Journal of Nutrition* 84 (October 2000): 417–27.

Shulman, Gerald I. "Cellular mechanisms of insulin resistance." *Journal of Clinical Investigation* 106:2 (July 15, 2000): 171–76.

Taylor, Valerie and Glenda MacQueen. "Associations Between Bipolar Disorder and Metabolic Syndrome: A Review." *Journal of Clinical Psychiatry* 67:7 (July 2006):1034–41.

Wood, Philip A. *How Fat Works.* Boston: Harvard University Press, 2006.

Yaffe, Kristine, Alka Kanaya, Karla Lindquist, Eleanor M. Simonsick, Tamara Harris, Ronald I. Shorr, Frances A. Tylavsky, and Anne B. Newman. "The Metabolic Syndrome, Inflammation, and Risk of Cognitive Decline." *Journal of the American Medical Association* 292:18 (November 10, 2004): 2237–42.

Young, Deborah, Patricia A. Lawlor, Paola Leone, Michael Dragunow, and Matthew J. During. "Environmental enrichment inhibits spontaneous apoptosis, prevents seizures and is neuroprotective." *Nature Medicine* 5 (April 1999): 448–53.

Index